Hypnofasting Program Guide

A Practical Plan to Lose Weight and
Control Type 2 Diabetes.

Joseph A. Onesta
Hypnofastingprogram.com Hypnofastingsolution.com

Hypnofasting Program Guide:

A Practical Plan to Lose Weight and Control Type 2 Diabetes

Joseph A. Onesta

ISBN: 978-1-7361870-1-2

First Printing: November 2020

Integrity HPI

Human Performance Improvement

www.intrgrityhpi.com

www.hypnofastingsolution.com

For valuable supplemental resources, including a PDF of the Supplemental Materials section with live internet links, visit, www.hypnofastingprogram.com.

To find a certified Hypnofasting Program Hypnotist, please visit www.hypnofastingprogram.com

If you are a clinical hypnotist and would like to be certified in The Hypnofasting Program, please visit www.hypnofastingsolution.com.

Who should read this book?

The Hypnofasting Program provides practical ways of addressing common key causes of obesity and type 2 diabetes.

If you struggle with your weight, you need this book. These days obesity is justifiably considered a disease. But simply applying the label without addressing the cause only perpetuates the problem. Obesity is the symptom, not the cause of the real disease, metabolic syndrome.

Labeling type 2 diabetes as a chronic and progressive disease is only half the story. Diabetes can be chronic and progressive if all we do is medically mitigate the symptom of high blood sugar but fail to address what causes the body to develop insulin resistance. The progression of type 2 diabetes can be controlled and even reversed.

I was both obese and diabetic and now I am neither. In the epilogue of this book, I confess, "When I began my own journey, I was completely alone, skeptical, and scared. I worried that it would not work. I was afraid that I would somehow do something stupid and further damage my health. It was frightening to learn that my health and wellness were in my hands and were not the sole auspices of my physician."

Your health and wellness belong in *your* hands, not only those of your doctor. I have taken all the critical material that I had to learn during my own recovery and have created The Hypnofasting Program, an easy-to-implement, stage-by-stage plan you can use to lose weight and/or gain control of type 2 diabetes.

Table of Contents

Chapter 1
It Happened One Day

"The doctor says you are diabetic, so watch what you eat." That was in 2004. The person on the other end of the phone was not my doctor, but just someone who worked in her office. We had just moved to Pittsburgh from Los Angeles. I was shocked. I had not expected anything like this news.

"What does that mean?" I asked.

"You're diabetic. Watch what you eat."

"You haven't answered my question. What should I eat?"

"I do not know, but they have classes over at the hospital. You can call over there."

"I'd like to speak with the doctor, please."

"She's not in." Then almost reluctantly, "I can make an appointment for you."

I hung up. My first reaction was an internal rant about a doctor who had an office worker call me and deliver such a message instead of doing it herself. I would be damned if I would make an appointment with that doctor again, ever.

My second reaction was to simply dismiss the call completely. I could not process it. Call the hospital and ask for what? What did it mean to be diabetic? How did I get diabetes? This was life-changing news, and I had no more room for any more change. I just ignored it for a year until I found another doctor and had another physical.

My new doctor also used the "D" word. He said that diabetes was a "chronic and progressive" condition and that I could slow down the progression of the disease if I lost weight. (Internal eye-roll—I admit it openly. How many times had I heard a doctor tell me to lose weight? It was literally the cure for virtually any complaint I had.) I let him know that weight was a constant struggle for me, and I needed a bit more from him on exactly how to do that.

"Diet and exercise," he said with a shrug of the shoulders. I could almost hear him thinking, *Duh...*

It was a moment of resignation for me. I had no idea what more I could do to lose weight. I had tried everything. I had led a lifetime of dieting. I spent thousands of dollars on supplements, diet shakes, home exercise equipment, and gym memberships. I had also wasted hours and hours with nutritionists, diet experts, and personal trainers.

I accepted the appointment with the hospital nutritionist. Believe it or not, I enjoyed meeting with her. She told me to eat smaller meals every two hours to level my blood sugar. I liked that. That is a lot better than starving myself. I already knew what the food pyramid said: I just had to snack every two hours in small amounts. Eat all day? I am in!

For over nearly fifteen years, I accepted the gradual progression of diabetes as a fact of life. After all, my doctor described diabetes as both chronic and progressive. I continued to follow the standard advice fairly closely. Sure, I diverged once in a while. No one, after all, is perfect. I faithfully took my medications and saw my doctor regularly. Year by year, my diabetes only got worse.

I lived with it. I did not become truly alarmed when my A1c (a three-month average of blood glucose levels) results were above 9. They had never been that high before! This meant that over a three-month period, my medications, my diet, and my activity levels were not sufficient to keep my blood sugar levels under control. My body was going crazy, and my doctor was advising a third medication before requiring insulin.

I began watching a lot of YouTube videos. These, it must be said, are not the best source of scientific research, but they are accessible, and I am pretty good at sorting through false information. One of the early videos I watched was by Dr. Jason Fung, who presented a different model of obesity and insulin resistance. He cited a lot of scientific research, which I ended up reading. His assertions made sense. His arguments were supported by evidence. He recommended a reduced carbohydrate diet and intermittent fasting. Why not? What did I have to lose?

I admit that the thought of "fasting" was abhorrent. And the thought of redesigning my diet without relying on carbohydrates was frightening. I began increasing the time between eating. At first, I made only small changes. I aggressively tested my blood because one of my medications could cause low blood sugar. As time passed and my blood glucose levels decreased, my energy levels increased. I felt encouraged to make even greater changes.

I had experienced symptoms of low blood sugar twice, and I had to gradually cut down on my diabetes medications. Within eight weeks, I was off medications entirely. Now, my blood glucose levels and my A1c are normal…not even prediabetic…normal. I have lost more than about a hundred pounds and counting. I have more energy. I think more clearly. My knees no longer hurt. I sleep better. And I have a whole new wardrobe.

As a clinical hypnotist, I also used self-hypnosis and exchanged sessions with colleagues to help me manage the process and stay motivated. The very idea of a low-carbohydrate diet and fasting, of all things, was unthinkable, and hypnosis and some mindfulness practice made it comparatively easy.

"The Hypnofasting Program" grew out of my experience with combining a low-carb diet and intermittent fasting, and my realization that the amount of information one needs to make informed decisions would be daunting for most people. I had to face those challenges alone. Now, you do not have to.

Since designing the program, I have worked with clients who have achieved either significant weight loss, more controlled diabetes, or both.

This book provides the basic information—which comes from licensed healthcare professionals—about a low carb/high healthy-fat diet and intermittent fasting in a gradual sequence that is easy to digest and easy to incorporate into your life. It also delivers some extremely helpful mindset strategies to make the changes easier to manage. But to get the most out of The Hypnofasting Program, you should work with a program-trained hypnotist and coach. Information about finding a qualified program hypnotist can be found on the program website: www.hypnofastingprogram.com.

It must be said that I am neither a physician, nutritionist, nor a licensed mental-health counselor. I am a consumer, a former diabetic, and a success story. I am also a clinical hypnosis practitioner who has researched this material primarily for my own consumption but also for my clients. However, nothing contained in this guide is intended as medical advice. You should keep your doctor apprised of changes in your lifestyle.

Whether you choose to work with a hypnotist or not, the practical information in this book will be useful. However, working with a hypnotist trained in this program will provide you with both the support of hypnosis and the practical and motivational coaching that a hypnotist can provide.

Joseph A. Onesta

Chapter 2
Obesity, Insulin Resistance, and Diabetes

If you are obese, it can be argued that you have some degree of "insulin resistance." What that generally means is that you may use more insulin to regulate blood glucose than people who are not obese. Type 2 diabetes is an extreme form of insulin resistance. Some diabetics must take one medication, while others might take two. Some diabetics literally have to inject insulin into their bodies to have enough insulin to do the job.

The essential problem is that diabetes treatment focuses on the removal of glucose, (sugar) from the blood. The process of removing glucose from the blood actually causes obesity. Obesity is not the problem, as in, "Lose weight and you will control your diabetes." If there is no other reason for your obesity, there has been so much glucose in your blood that your liver had no alternative but to convert it into fat.

The Carbohydrate-Insulin Model

When I first was diagnosed with type 2 diabetes, the doctor told me diabetes was a chronic and progressive illness. I could control the progression of the disease with diet, exercise, and a pill. He did not explain the diet in detail but sent me to a nutritionist. He gave me a prescription for Metformin and told me to lose weight and get more exercise.

I had been hearing the admonition to lose weight and exercise more for years. After countless attempts at altering my diet and thousands of wasted dollars on consultants, trainers, supplements, and gym memberships, all my efforts to lose weight and keep it off were disappointing. Frustrating is a better word. After a while, I learned to live with being fat and accepted feeling both helpless and guilty for it.

The meeting with the nutritionist was typical. Her advice was the standard offered at the time: I should get about 60% of my calories from carbohydrates and eat smaller meals more frequently—every two hours or so, to keep my blood sugar levels stable. At the time, it was what the "science" said, but frankly, it was the exact opposite of what I should do.

Here is why: the default fuel of the body is glucose. When we eat carbohydrates, our body converts them almost immediately into glucose, causing our blood sugar levels to rise easily and quickly. Complex carbohydrates might do this a bit more slowly, but they still do it. No matter how complex a carbohydrate may be, it is still a carbohydrate.

Insulin, secreted by the pancreas, is what the body uses to maintain healthy blood glucose levels. When we eat carbohydrates, blood glucose rises, triggering the production of insulin. (It is not the only trigger for insulin production, but it is the one that we can measure easily.) The more carbohydrates we consume, the more insulin is needed to maintain healthy blood sugar levels.

Insulin takes the glucose from the blood, deposits what we need in our muscles, and sends the excess to the liver. The liver stores excess glucose in two forms. It stores a short-term quantity as glycogen. Short-term glycogen basically is what your liver thinks you will need for the day. (Most people get close to that many carbohydrates in a bowl of cereal with 2% milk. Or let's face facts, in a single double-decaf, nonfat latte with a squirt of caramel.) Over time, constant and consistent excess glucose overwhelms our system, and we need more insulin to do the job. The cells receiving the glucose are full and, for lack of a better metaphor, cannot take another bite. That is called "insulin resistance."

Thus, more and more glucose is forced into the liver until we cannot produce enough insulin to do the job. Then we are labeled as diabetic and are given medications to force the liver into submission and increase insulin.

In normal conditions, when blood glucose levels go down, the liver releases glycogen as glucose into the blood to keep levels normal, and, in reality, we do not need to eat for energy.

When the short-term stores are not consumed because we keep eating and snacking throughout the day, the liver takes excess glycogen and converts it into fat. The process is called *de novo lipogenesis*, big words for "making fat."

The fat is first stored around our organs and then in fat cells around the body. If we can see the fat on our bodies, we can be relatively certain that there is fat around our organs. Has your doctor ever used the words "fatty liver"?

It is not enough to reduce calories to lose weight. A reduced calorie diet will work temporarily, but the consumption of fewer calories leads to natural adjustments in metabolism, making our bodies function on fewer calories. That is the opposite of what we want.

But, if we understand more about how our bodies process nutrients, we can give our body what it needs to do what we want it to do. That is, burn our stores of fat and manage blood glucose in a healthy way. If you have type 2 diabetes, the process may take some time. In the long run, however, it is well worth the effort and time required.

According to this model, to lose weight and control our blood sugar at the same time, we need to do the following:

- Consume less sugar and foods that readily convert to sugar (glucose) in our bodies, i.e., carbohydrates.

- Eat less frequently, allowing our bodies to use up the glucose in our cells and the daily glycogen stores in the liver so that it is not being converted into fat.

- Extend the time between eating to allow our bodies to use up all the glycogen stores and begin accessing the stored fat and use it as energy.

- Provide our bodies the proper nutrients, sufficient calories, and proper activity levels to perform efficiently and maintain a healthy metabolism.

  Establish a sustainable lifestyle so that our bodies stabilize at our target weight or condition.

For a more extensive explanation of this model, see "A New Paradigm of Insulin Resistance." (Fung, 2017)

If You Are Diabetic...

If you have been diagnosed with type 2 diabetes or prediabetes, you are probably taking medications to keep your blood sugar levels in check. It is extremely important that you aggressively and consistently monitor your blood glucose levels because your medications have been designed to control those levels. As you begin to control your own blood glucose levels through diet, activity, and fasting, you run the risk of experiencing low blood sugar levels that can be quite dangerous.

Low blood sugar levels can result in unconsciousness and even death. If you are using insulin or taking medications that may lower your blood sugar levels, and you follow this plan, testing your blood glucose frequently is of the utmost importance. You should keep food or juice handy to quickly counteract low blood sugar levels, should that become necessary. Therefore, you need to be able to easily recognize the symptoms of low blood sugar levels. (Symptoms)

Your physician should be involved in any changes to your medication levels. It is likely that those medications will need to be adjusted as you progress through the program. Know that rapid changes may not be reflected in your A1c results until you have seen consistently reduced levels for three months.

If You Are Vegetarian or Vegan...

The principles of hypnofasting present a diet that relies heavily on increasing protein and healthy fat and decreasing reliance on carbohydrates. Vegetarians and vegans can benefit from intermittent fasting but may have difficulty achieving the reduced levels of carbohydrates and an increased healthy fat that are essential for the program. Despite popular recommendations, science does not back up the healthfulness of polyunsaturated fats (most cooking oils from seeds), especially after hydrogenation. (Knobbe) Additionally, saturated fats have been unscientifically demonized in our society, and scientific evidence indicates the opposite of what we have been taught. (Teicholz, 2015) Use of vegetable, corn, or any of the seed oils—including partially or fully hydrogenated (trans fat) versions—is not recommended in The Hypnofasting Program.

As a vegetarian or vegan, your ability to apply the principles of The Hypnofasting Program will require more work on your part because many plant-based sources of protein also come with significant levels of carbohydrates. If you are going to consume soy or gluten products as your main source of protein, at least consider only organic sources.

Vegetarian and vegan sources of natural fat are limited. Many of the health promises put forth about polyunsaturated oils lack clear scientific benefit, and deleterious or negative consequences of relying on these oils have often been demonstrated. Extra virgin olive oil is a monounsaturated fat. Avocado oil contains saturated and both mono- and polyunsaturated fats. Vegan sources of saturated fat are coconut and red palm oil, which are solid at room temperature.

You, of course, can eat what you want. The decision is yours, and you should make it with the best possible information.

I am not some carnivore mocker of vegans and vegetarians. In fact, I was a lacto-ovo vegetarian for nearly twenty years. In 1992, I saw a nutritionist to lose weight. We followed the traditional reduced-calorie, low-fat advice still used by many today. I lost about three hundred pounds. It was about then I opted for vegetarianism, as I was not eating much meat anyway, and I was rather put off by industrial husbandry.

As advised, my diet relied heavily on grains, vegetables, and restricted fat. I only consumed the white of the eggs for protein. (No yolks because of the cholesterol.) Dairy products occupied only a small, almost negligible, portion of my diet. At the time, the supermarket shelves were filled with products labeled "fat free." I even became quite good at baking all sorts of delicious things without fat.

After achieving my goal and staying on the diet but no longer counting calories, the thirty pounds I lost gradually became the hundred pounds I gained. After that, no matter how hard I tried, I could not lose that weight again following that diet. I settled in at almost three hundred pounds.

Based on my own research into this issue, I now fully attribute both my obesity and my diabetes to that diet and the subsequent low-fat, high-carb lifestyle. I do not blame the doctor or the nutritionist. They were following the USDA recommendations at the time, recommendations which are still being proffered. (Choose) I am not suggesting that everyone will have the same results as I did. However, I will point out that since the 1980s, our society has followed the USDA guidelines, and both obesity and diabetes are evident in epidemic proportions. (Teicholz, 2019)

A Real Food Movement

It is only fair to point out that I stress real food as part of The Hypnofasting Program. That means buying whole ingredients, planning meals, and cooking. Those ingredients should be as natural, in season, and organic as you can afford. Hypnofasters have to learn a lot about what they put in their bodies. That is why hypnofasting exists! You, of course, can choose to embrace whatever elements of this program best serve your needs. If you find yourself fearful of cooking, please open your mind to the possibility of spending more time in the kitchen. If you frequent restaurants for convenience, consider gradually setting aside an increasing amount of time for food preparation. Increasing the quality of your life is well worth the effort.

Joseph A. Onesta

Chapter 3
A New Normal

The Hypnofasting Program is not merely about reaching a target weight or stabilizing your blood glucose. It is more than that. Way more. It is about establishing a new pattern of attitude and behavior, a new lifestyle. In fact, it is about creating a new "normal" in your life.

I have heard countless people say, "I wish I could be like so-and-so. They can eat whatever they want and never gain a pound." It is not a fair comparison, but my guess is that if we compared apples to apples, we would find significant differences in the things they want to eat and the frequency with which they eat them. That is what The Hypnofasting Program is all about: changing what you want, not merely losing a few pounds.

Also, do not be envious of people who eat a lot of junk food and still appear fit. Outward appearances can be deceiving. Despite looking fit, many of them have fat stored inside their abdomen around the organs behind the abdominal wall—a condition labeled Thin on the Outside, but Fat on the Inside (TOFI). These unfortunate folks are often ignorant of their risk for negative health consequences, such as heart attack or stroke, which are as great as those of us who display obesity for all to see. (David)

Remember, above all, this one simple thing: the way we lived before we started hypnofasting resulted in the very thing we now want to change. We have to think and behave differently for the rest of our lives to change the rest of our lives.

Many people are looking for an easy way out. They want a magic pill, a superfood, a piece of equipment, a prepackaged meal, a convenient product, or a dietary supplement that will resolve their problem. These products represent billion-dollar industries, and there is no end to them because none of them actually work over the long term.

The Hypnofasting Program is designed for permanent change because it addresses both the mind and the body, thus facilitating the necessary adjustments to one's lifestyle. It is not just a plan; it is a program for change.

There are people who say they want to lose weight or control their diabetes, but what they really mean is, if you will forgive the cliché, they want to have their cake and eat it, too. They do not want to give up eating what they want now. They want a better life without actually working to change the one they have. Well, this is the only one we have right now. Let's stop dreaming and work to change it.

We know that restricted calorie diets do not work in the long term and may well cause increasing damage to our bodies. We know that dieters lose and gain repeatedly and eventually just give up. We know that exercise does not burn enough calories to make a real difference, and any progress is not permanent. Have you ever seen a reunion show for winners of *The Biggest Loser*? I challenge you. Go on YouTube and search. You will see that those miraculous changes were not miraculous at all. Most of them were at best temporary, like a mirage.

What Is "Normal?"

Your mind-body naturally settles into what is normal for you. Right now, what you see in the mirror, the numbers that appear on your scale or your glucometer, is what is normal for you. It is where you have settled in, and the natural propensity of your brain-body is to return to this condition after any temporary change.

Some of the changes we make in The Hypnofasting Program will be temporary. When you make decisions about what you choose to eat, you may, for a while, make more drastic choices in order to achieve your goals. However, in The Hypnofasting Program, we work to sustain a new condition long enough to reset what the brain-body considers normal. You may choose, once again, to occasionally eat a food you have eliminated during the program. But the one thing that will not change is that you will always make informed decisions about what you eat.

"Everyone in my family is fat. What chance do I have?" Some suggest that body weight, or the occurrence of diabetes, is genetically determined. Truth is, your obesity is more likely because of the food culture shared by your family than your genetic makeup.

We recognize that genes allow for certain potential conditions. It was once hoped that genetic modification might actually cure diseases. As it turns out, we do not have to actually modify your genes; we can turn them on and off. The science of "epigenetics" demonstrates that the function of genes can be influenced by their environment, indicating that lasting change is possible. To learn more about epigenetics, read *The Biology of Belief.* (Lipton)

It takes sustained changes over a long period of time for your brain-body to accept and settle into a new condition of normalcy. Once that happens, you will have more wiggle room and, by the time that happens, due to the practical and psychological changes you have made, you should be far less inclined to abuse that flexibility and actually become a bit more like so-and-so who eats whatever they want without gaining a pound.

Why Hypnosis?

The Hypnofasting Program is hypnosis-facilitated lifestyle change to lose weight and control type 2 diabetes. But why bring up hypnosis at all if the practical information in this book will do the job?

You can, of course, follow a low-carb, high-healthy fat diet combined with intermittent fasting all on your own. Working with a qualified Hypnofasting Program hypnotist, however, provides two distinct advantages. First, you have a coach to answer your questions, guide you through the process, and work with you to resolve any glitches, even tailoring the program to your specific needs.

Of equal if not greater importance is that you gain the power of *changing your mind.*

All change, even positive change, creates stress. Some of us can maintain motivation and emotional strength throughout the stress of change and do it without help. Most of us, however, need support, strategies, and tools for adapting to the changes we want to make.

Hypnosis is not magic, but it sometimes feels that way. Hypnosis is a way of getting new information to your unconscious mind so that it can make better informed decisions. Your unconscious mind decides all your automatic behaviors, thoughts, emotions, and reactions. Hypnosis allows our unconscious mind to accept the changes our conscious minds want to make.

Think of it this way: many people want to quit smoking, knowing that smoking will shorten their lives, lead to limited lung function and possibly cancer, yet part of them still believes that smoking is useful for relaxation, perhaps enjoyment, or what-have-you. So, they continue to smoke despite their conscious understanding. This is the reason hypnosis is the most successful method of kicking the habit.

Hypnosis:

- Reduces anxiety
- Boosts the immune system

- Helps fight cravings
- Facilitates acceptance
- Increases motivation and commitment
- Combats emotional eating
- Provides positive self-soothing
- Builds resolve
- Gets us through tough times
- Helps change the way we experience life
- Feels great

How to Use This Book

This is not really a self-help manual, but you can use it that way because it contains an easy-to-follow practical plan. I and trained hypnotists use this plan as a practical guide to help our clients, while working with them using hypnosis. You can, of course, read and follow the material as you like; but to get the most out of this book and have help with whatever pitfalls you might encounter, find a hypnotist who has been trained in the program. A list of trained hypnotists is available at www.hypnofastingprogram.com. Your hypnotist will invite you to participate in our Facebook Group where you can ask questions, share your experiences, exchange recipes, and connect with other hypnofasters.

If you try to integrate The Hypnofasting Program with a restricted-calorie diet, you will fail. You will likely stall prior to reaching your goal and/or you will quickly regain the weight or increase your insulin resistance thereafter. You have got to give up the calories-in versus calories-out model. You have to stop counting or even being concerned about eating too many calories. Some hypnofasters, at one point or another, actually worry that they are not getting enough calories because they feel satisfied and seem to be eating less than they did before joining the program.

Any information in this book directed toward type 2 diabetics applies to prediabetics as well. If you are taking medications for diabetes, you will need to test your blood glucose levels several times a day. Get a blood glucose meter if you do not already have one. Ask your doctor for a prescription for one or just go and buy one over the counter.

There is a subtle difference between the labels "mind-body" and "brain-body," though the labels often overlap. I consider the brain-body to be mechanical, while the mind-body includes perceptions and emotions. There is mutual influence between the mind-body and the brain-body.

The book is organized in stages. Complete one stage before proceeding to the next. You determine the rate in which you progress through the program, but a week or two at any one stage should be sufficient. The ultimate goal of The Hypnofasting Program is for you to gain enough understanding and discipline to continue learning and advancing your health on your own.

If you are working with a certified Hypnofasting Program hypnotist, I urge you to not read ahead but agree with your hypnotist about proceeding to the next stage. The topics covered in each stage have been carefully designed to address changes that when taken all at once may seem overwhelming, but when taken step-by-step are easier to accommodate and accomplish.

While the information contained here is good and valid as of the date of publication, science is always advancing. Stay informed. Keep researching and rethinking. As Dr. Ken Berry often says, "Do not believe me. Read the research yourself."

The stages described in the process revolve around the gradual process of incorporating a diet decreasingly dependent on carbohydrates and developing a pattern of intermittent fasting for both weight loss and control of type 2 diabetes. Each stage builds upon the last.

In this program, you will encounter the words "keto," "ketogenic," and "LCHF," the acronym for low-carb/high-fat. Simply, the keto or ketogenic diet is a method of choosing what is consumed so that the body uses body fat and begins to burn ketones instead of solely glucose sugar as fuel. To stick to a ketogenic diet, one eats very few carbohydrates per day. A LCHF diet shares many qualities with a ketogenic diet but is less restrictive. A LCHF diet can more easily be scaled to individual preferences and more easily avoid processed foods that have been labeled "keto" merely because of the low carbohydrates but may be inadvisable for other reasons.

I have tried to keep the supplemental materials to this book as unacademic as possible to make the material readily accessible to just about anyone who reads or watches videos. I have chosen to reference or suggest these materials because they appeared to me to be particularly credible or useful.

All of the source material for this program and the supplemental materials referenced are listed in the back of the book under "Supplemental Materials." When I wish to point your attention to one of these sources, usually for supplemental videos or articles, the reference will be followed in parentheses by the first word of the citation so you can find it easily on the alphabetized list. When a single author or source is listed more than once, the parenthetical citation will include a distinguishing element, like the date of publication or a word or two from the title. Online sources include source URL to help you access the materials. For a free, easy-to-click, live-link version of the supplemental materials list visit our website:

www.hypnofastingprogram.com.

Watch the sourced videos! Learning is a key part of this program. Watch the videos. Read the articles. Look up the material.

If you choose to follow this program, you will follow a low-carbohydrate diet and utilize intermittent fasting. If you are not sure about making this move, do your research. I strongly urge you to investigate and educate yourself beyond the materials included in this program, which, in some cases, fly in the face of standard practices for losing weight and diabetes control. Your knowledge and understanding are your power and impetus to sustained change, and they are the only way you can proceed with confidence.

Barbarians at the Gate

Because the low-carb, high-fat diet goes against the strongly defended status-quo recommendations of government agencies, Nina Teicholz points out, we are like "barbarians at the gate." There is a growing number of both professional and laypeople examining and reexamining the assumptions many of us have simply accepted as true. For many reasons, many are invested in the status quo, and the mounting evidence against their recommendations threatens them. Expect to receive some opposition from friends, family, and perhaps even your doctor to the choices you might make by participating in this program. The principles of this program may be new and unfamiliar to many doctors who likely have the absolute best of intentions. Most physicians receive extraordinarily little education in nutrition; even if they did, what they might be taught is likely based on very questionable nutrition science. (Teicholz, 2015)

This questionable science, promoted by a dynamic nutritional theorist named Ancel Keys, has been embraced by both political and social organizations. Many of those who legitimately and scientifically opposed the theories of Ancel Keys risked and lost their careers to do so. (Teicholz, 2019)

While I urge you to involve your physician in your utilization of this program, and to make no changes to your prescribed treatments without your doctor's full knowledge, I also urge you to do your research and learn about the decisions you are making. Do not just believe me, but learn, so that you know you are making the right decisions for yourself.

I was incredibly lucky. My doctor listened to me when I presented my evidence. I brought real evidence. I presented my doctor with a spreadsheet of my blood glucose readings and my fasting hours for four months. Additionally, my blood work indicated an A1c reading of 5.4 when the previous one was near 10!

"The numbers don't lie" was all he said. I could tell he remained skeptical as I knew he would. He needed to see my change last. He is a good doctor. I like him because he at least listens to me. But if he had formidably opposed my informed decisions, I would have found a new doctor.

Dr. Berry, in his book *Lies My Doctor Told Me*, offers some wonderful suggestions for working with your doctor. This may well mean bringing your fasting journals the next time you visit your doctor. I used a spreadsheet to present my data to my doctor. Your records and progress will help your doctor understand this program better.

Counting the Cost

Following this program is a choice. You will always be in control of what you do, the changes you make, and which parts of this program work best for you. The more you embrace, the more dramatic the change will be. The more aggressively you adopt the changes, the more quickly you will see results. But you can, indeed, take the program very slowly and still eventually see results.

We will be following a LCHF diet for the purpose of controlling insulin both for weight loss and for better control of type 2 diabetes. This means gradually changing what you eat.

We will also employ the practice of intermittent fasting. This means eating at controlled times until you adjust. Dr. Maggs has an informative video that presents the "Pros and Cons of Intermittent Fasting." (Maggs, Pros and Cons)

Your education is key for several reasons. First, if you understand what you are doing, you will be better at deciding what you want to do. Second, you will face opposition and need to know how to cope with it. Third, you will likely need to educate your physician on the process and its value.

Joseph A. Onesta

Chapter 4
Stage One

In this first stage, we will primarily focus on getting ready for change. Please remain in this stage for at least a week. Since I do not know what you know, nor do I know what you think, it is best for us to proceed methodically. In this stage, we will cover some basic information, learn how to track our progress, and make a single major change in the way we eat.

Macronutrients

We can conveniently break down all food into three categories, called "macronutrients." They are protein, carbohydrates, and fats. Very few foods actually fit snugly into a single category. Most deliver more than one macronutrient in varying percentages. We are concerned about the main or dominant macronutrient. Bread, for example, is primarily a carbohydrate but contains some protein in the form of gluten and often contains some fat.

Critically, each macronutrient is processed by the body differently and thus has a different effect on blood glucose and the consequential insulin secretion. This fact is also one of the essential reasons that reducing our understanding of weight to calories in versus calories out is doomed to failure. A fat calorie is not the same as a carbohydrate calorie. The sharpest insulin response is quickly triggered by carbohydrates. Proteins take a bit longer to digest and have a moderate effect on blood glucose and insulin. Fat causes the lowest degree of insulin response.

The "glycemic index" is a standardized list of the effects of different foods on blood glucose levels. The higher an item is ranked on the list, the greater the effect it has on blood glucose levels. The index can serve as a guide, but everyone is a little different. The experience of an individual may diverge from the list. Harvard Health has a website that introduces the glycemic index and lists the ranking of 100 common foods. (Harvard)

A well-planned LCHF diet is designed to provide the nutritional needs of your body while maintaining the lowest possible insulin response.

Hunger

No one likes to be hungry. Let's be honest—it does not feel good. Most of us feel hungry several times a day. Some of us feel hunger almost constantly.

I dare say that the majority of us have never *truly* been hungry. For most of us, the feeling of hunger is an interpretation of something, an experience, a thought, an emotion. In fact, we most often feel hunger as a matter of habit. That is, we get hungry when we think it is time to eat. Some of us constantly feel hungry because we have grown accustomed to grazing or snacking all day long.

In my youth, I had a friend who went with his church on a mission trip to an impoverished place. Upon his return, it was obvious that the trip had affected him. He had grown more thoughtful and contemplative. I knew the trip had changed him. Prior to going, he had been very excited, but he returned with few stories of adventures.

As we sat in my family room, listening to music and talking about school, I broached the subject. "You haven't said much about your trip. Tell me about it."

He had a few stories, but he seemed like he did not really want to talk about it. Then he said, "I will never again be able to say I am starving." Tearfully, he told me of meeting people who really did not have food. "Those pictures you see of kids with distended stomachs on television—they're true. They are starving, for real! Having the munchies is not starving. It is not even hungry."

What we call hunger is really just an urge to eat that begins with multiple possible triggers. It is an automatic response, and though our bodies may not be hungry, we feel hungry. That feeling may range from simply the desire to eat to a feeling of frantic urgency.

We feel hungry if the clock is approaching our normal mealtimes. We feel hungry when our blood sugar drops. The feeling of hunger can be triggered by the smells of certain foods or the sight of other appetizing items. Even the thoughts and memories we have can trigger feelings of hunger or cravings. We may feel hungry in response to certain emotions. We think we are hungry if our stomach growls a bit.

Over the last fifty years, our society has shifted from eating three square meals a day to eating those meals and casually snacking in between. Many people graze throughout the day. The result is almost a constant feeling of hunger. As a society, we are almost always ready to eat, and when we are not eating, we feel a bit hungry. I have had clients tell me that they had no idea what it meant to feel full or satisfied.

There was a time when children were routinely denied a snack after school because it might "ruin" their dinner. Now, more commonly, kids snack to tide themselves over until dinner. What a difference!

Real hunger is not merely having an empty stomach. In fact, throughout history, human stomachs have often routinely been empty.

From early humans who ate only when they found or successfully hunted food, to well within the last hundred years, people simply lived with an empty stomach until food was available. I keep thinking about those old movies when farmhands stopped working when the sound of a triangle bell told them that supper was ready.

As a result of industrial agriculture, processed, prepackaged foods, the emergence of fast and convenient foods, and the flood of television commercials promoting a myriad of snacks and easy-to-prepare processed foods, American society has been trained to snack and do it frequently. We have been trained to eat all the time. The more we eat, the more money they make.

One of the arguments in favor of the industrialization of food is that we need the food to feed a rising population. Truth be told, upwards of 40% of the food produced in the United States is wasted and ends up in the landfill. (USDA) Perhaps if we consumed healthier food in more reasonable quantities, we would not have such waste. At that rate, we could easily decrease farm intensity and sponsor more organic and humanely produced food.

Instead of sitting down to a home-cooked, whole-food dinner, we are carting little Brittany off to soccer and young Jimmy to martial arts, handing them bags of chips, cookies, yogurt packs, and pudding snacks just tiding them over until, on the way home, we hand them a bag of something we picked up at a drive-through.

Sadly, much of what we consume in the form of processed foods is nutritionally lacking, or the enriched nutrients are not well processed by the body. People in modern society are often overfed and undernourished. Overweight people are not lacking sufficient fuel. In fact, they have excess. That is why they are fat. But they may well be lacking in nutrition, and their bodies may have become less efficient because of the lack of nutrient dense food and sedentary lifestyles.

We have to learn to recognize the difference between real hunger and merely feeling hungry. The feelings of hunger pass quickly. They come and go like waves and are nothing more than a response to some stimulus that tells us it is time to eat. Feeling hungry is most often just a feeling and not a biological necessity.

When you feel hungry, take a moment to observe the feeling. Where is it in your body? We associate hunger with an empty stomach, but you might well be surprised about where the feeling of hunger resides in your body. It may be in your stomach, but often it is sensed elsewhere. Sometimes it is felt in the mouth, and this may mean you are more thirsty than hungry. A glass of water may be all it takes to quench the urge. A sense of hunger may be felt in the chest, the hands, around the temples, as a pressure in the forehead, or even low in the gut. It may even be sensed as a nagging thought or emotional urge.

Once you find it, just observe it for a while. Do not judge it as good or bad. Do not try getting away from it by putting something into your mouth. Do not let it make you frantic. Just observe it. What does it do? Does it change in intensity? How about in its urgency? Does it disappear?

Carbohydrate Hunger

When we eat carbohydrates, our blood glucose rapidly increases, signaling our pancreas to produce insulin. In the presence of that insulin, if our muscles have what they need, the excess glucose is removed from the bloodstream and stored in the liver. As the insulin removes the glucose, we experience a drop in blood sugar that triggers our brain to signal the feeling of hunger. If we were completely healthy, our blood sugar would not fluctuate so dramatically, and we would actually feel less hungry. We might even know what it means to have an empty stomach while still feeling satisfied. Imagine that!

All carbohydrates, both simple and complex, cause a marked increase in blood glucose. While whole grains have more fiber and might slightly slow down this process, it still takes place, and the change is still dramatic. Eating foods that are high in carbohydrates results in feeling hungry more frequently and often more intensely because a drop in blood sugar, especially after a sharp spike, sends signals to the brain that things are changing. Hunger, sleepiness, listlessness, and sugar cravings can result from the rapid drop in blood glucose that is affected by your own body responding with insulin.

This cycle needs to be interrupted. As we proceed through the program, you may well notice a marked difference in the above-mentioned side effects as your blood sugar levels stabilize and your diet becomes less dependent on the foods that cause rapid blood glucose spikes. You will certainly feel less hungry.

Hunger and Satiety

Hunger and satiety are functions of two hormones. "Ghrelin" tells you it is time to eat and "leptin" makes you feel satisfied. (Magee) The key with these hormones is that their goal is "homeostasis," or a return to normal. If you have been overweight and/or over-consuming high-carbohydrate foods, these hormones recognize the change and attempt to trigger hunger or satiety in hopes of maintaining what is normal for you.

It might surprise you to know that overriding a hormone is not an easy thing to do, but we do it all the time. If we eat when we are not hungry—say, to try something, taste something, or to indulge in a special treat—we are overriding leptin. If you have ever finished your portion or plate of food even though you no longer felt hunger, you have overridden leptin. Doing that takes willpower.

We suppress desires with what we call willpower, sometimes associating the objects of our desires with unpleasant things or forsaking one desire to obtain another. Establishing a new mind-body balance, in other words, a new normal, takes time and effort. The effort is exercising our willpower, something you already do without knowing it. This is where hypnosis comes in handy because we need to change our automatic assumptions about what is normal for us.

Critical to a healthy balance of ghrelin and leptin is establishing and maintaining a healthy gut microbiome. Many medications and, believe it or not, many processed foods have a detrimental effect on the important microorganisms in the gut. Wheat gluten, for example, causes microbiome disturbance whether or not a person is sensitive or has celiac disease. Taking an antibiotic medication can have devastating effects on the good microbes in your gut. And many serious conditions like inflammatory bowel disease, liver cancer, and metabolic syndrome have been linked to microbiome imbalance. (Perlmutter)

As we proceed with the program, you may notice changes in your bowel habits or movements. If you have been unhealthy for a long time, or if you have taken antibiotics, it might be a good idea to use a probiotic supplement. Increasing the fiber content of your diet can also help you cultivate a healthy microbiome.

Your Natural Fast

Unless you eat in your sleep, you already fast every day. Fasting is natural, easy, and important. We call this our "natural" fast. Unfortunately, many of us have cultivated the habit of eating from the time we wake until the time we go to bed. This means that, except for the time we are actually asleep, we are almost constantly stimulating the production of insulin, especially if we are snacking on carbohydrate-laden foods.

From this point forward in our program, we will track our natural fast, and as we proceed, we will expand it so that your body can use up the glucose, glycogen, and ultimately the fat it has stored around your organs and elsewhere on your body. In doing this, we also naturally train our bodies to require less insulin and even increase insulin sensitivity, virtually stalling diabetes and even reversing insulin resistance.

Whatever our natural fast is, chances are that it is either insufficient or inefficient to manage our consumption of food. That is why we get fat. That is why some of us develop type 2 diabetes.

The Program Journal

Keeping a journal during the program is important so that we can understand where you are and what you eventually need to accomplish to achieve your goals. Keeping a journal has two main purposes in The Hypnofasting Program.

The first purpose of the journal is to set a baseline and record your progress in concrete terms. If you keep accurate records, you will see your progress and know that the program is working. You will then be able to better judge changes you need to make and when you have reached the stopping place from which you maintain the status quo long enough to convince your brain-body that you are establishing a new normal.

The second purpose is for you to become aware of the interrelated factors in your lifestyle that have contributed to your weight and/or your type 2 diabetes. If you understand these factors in the context of how your body functions, you will be able to make changes that are appropriate for you as an individual. Do not skimp on the journals. Do not put off completing them.

You can design your own forms or download the one I have designed in PDF format from www.hypnofastingprogram.com.

If you are working with a program hypnotist, they may want to occasionally review your journal. Please bring it with you to your sessions.

Whether you use the program journal provided on our website, www.hypnofastingprogram.com, or design your own, the important thing is that we record the necessary information. We need to know how long your daily natural fast is. That is, how many hours pass between your last bite the night before and your first bite the next day.

We also need to know when, what, and how much you eat each time you eat. No need to measure the quantities. If you eat a hamburger and fries, you have a visual amount in your mind; that is all we need for now. You would also include your beverages and condiments, such as ketchup, mayo, etc. In stage one, you can eat whatever you would normally eat in your normal quantities.

Make notes if you have any emotional side effects of eating. Anything from a feeling of relief to guilt about whatever. These are important to share with your hypnotherapist, and if you are attempting to work alone, you might want to consider working with a hypnotist.

If you are diabetic, we want to keep some additional information; most notably, test and record your blood glucose levels just before your first bite of the day and then take and record a second reading about two hours after you eat each meal. (No snacking between meals.) Notice when your sugar spikes more than thirty points above your fasting blood glucose reading. This might happen a lot at first. Compare the spikes to what you ate two hours before. Try to isolate the foods that cause the most precipitous jump in your blood sugar readings.

Your First Big Change

Perhaps it is due to our busy lives, perhaps it is because we graze more than eat specific meals, but many of us eat without thinking. In fact, with the very first bite, many people go into eating autopilot. We may be watching television, working at our computer, or just reading the back of the cereal box. Whatever we are doing, our minds are not really on the food. In other words, we are eating mindlessly.

Those days of grabbing something quickly, shoveling in fast food as you drive, or sitting in front of your television or computer while you munch must become a thing of the past. These activities lead to mindless eating. Have you ever discovered that you had cleaned your plate without realizing it?

While I have met a number of morbidly obese people who indeed eat comparatively little, the vast majority of them have no idea how much they actually eat. Sometimes they do not even remember eating, much less what they actually ate.

In order to eat more mindfully, we need to focus our attention on what we are eating, when we are eating it, and even *why* we are eating it. Take your time. Go bite by bite.

If you have prepared the food yourself, concentrate on the process and take note of the sight, smell, and textures of the ingredients. Notice and listen to the sound the knife makes on the cutting board, the sizzling bacon, the boiling pot.

Do not eat standing up. Choose an eating environment as free as possible from distraction or interruption. Take a moment to consider your meal. Pause before you begin eating. If it is your custom, say grace. If grace is not your custom, take a moment to change your mindset and prepare to eat. This is your intentional act to alert your body that you are eating. You are telling your body that this is the time to get those digestive processes in motion.

Notice the subtle aroma of the food as you bring it to your mouth, the temperature, texture, and flavor as you chew, and the physical sensations of swallowing completely before you take the next bite. This is known as "mindful eating."

Avoid "washing down" your bites with a beverage. You can drink, but it is separate from chewing a bit of food. Swallow your food before you sip. Notice the weight of the glass or cup, the slight pressure in your mouth as you sip, the temperature and flavor of your beverage, and the sensations of swallowing.

In other words, think about what you are doing!

Halfway through the meal, stop and reassess. Ask yourself if you still feel hungry or whether your sense of hunger has abated. How do you feel? Could you stop now? As your mind and body adjust, you may realize that your hunger was never as strong as you thought it was and that you can easily stop somewhere in the middle of the meal and not need to look for something else to eat.

If you emotionally need to finish your plate because that is the way you were raised, begin to serve yourself only half the amount you normally would. If, upon completion of that reduced portion, you would like a bit more, then take a bit more. But notice, again, what you are choosing to eat and why you are choosing it.

Take a moment to write several sentences in your journal about the meal. It can be anything from your feelings to your reaction to having tried something new.

Reflecting on these notes can help you identify patterns of thought and behavior that may be easy to change. Do you always clean your plate? Do you overfill your plate? Do you always reach for seconds? There are easy life-changing responses to these patterns of behavior. Make your hypnotist aware of these patterns.

Joseph A. Onesta

Chapter 5
Stage Two

Carbohydrates, Proteins, and Fats

The glycemic index, as mentioned earlier, gives us a good indication of how our blood sugar levels might react to different foods and is a valuable resource when we plan our meals, but we do not have to memorize the index to have a good, firm grasp on what causes blood sugar spikes.

As you know, there are only three main macronutrients: carbohydrates, proteins, and fats. Very few foods fit into only one of these categories. Most foods contain more than one macronutrient, so we choose to concern ourselves with generalized categories.

Refined sugar has no nutritive value whatsoever. But, when we think of carbohydrates, we may think of "sugar" because carbohydrate is the macronutrient most easily converted into glucose. Foods made mostly of grains—wheat, rice, barley, rye, corn, and oats—are sources mostly of carbohydrates. We then must also add sweet produce like fruit and beets. We also include root vegetables like potatoes, carrots, and yams. Most vegetables have some level of carbohydrate, but the biggest offenders are the starchy ones that often grow underground. Vegetables, not grains, that produce fruit above ground are comparatively low in carbohydrates and have less dramatic effects on blood glucose levels.

Legumes straddle the line between carbohydrates and proteins. While most beans have protein, for most hypnofasters, they are better considered a source of carbohydrate. Vegetarian and vegan hypnofasters have to balance these out as legumes for them may be a primary source of protein, but the carbohydrate content cannot be ignored.

Proteins are meat, seafood, eggs, and dairy products. Proteins have a less dramatic effect on blood glucose levels than do carbohydrates. Dairy, particularly liquid dairy, contains significant sugars in the form of lactose, and many dairy products are sweetened. Milk products that claim to be lactose-free do not have the lactose removed but rather enzymes added to aid in the digestion of lactose.

Sources of fat are olives, nuts, seeds, avocados, and whole dairy. Foods that are primary sources of fat have the least effect on blood glucose levels. But consider that fat generally comes with something else. Fat may come with protein, such as in the marbling of meat. It may come with carbohydrates, like in olives, nuts, and seeds.

These general concepts focus on whole foods. But processed or manufactured foods require some attention. Most manufactured foods contain a mixture of ingredients. Some of them are cheap fillers in order to make the processed foods more affordable to consumers while simultaneously more profitable for manufacturers. Often these filler foods come in the form of grains or grain byproducts. The next time you go to a restaurant, notice how much of the meal is made up of cheap carbohydrates, such as bread, pasta, potatoes, or rice.

In my youth, one of my closest friends was from Taiwan, and a bunch of us often went to a Chinese restaurant where we ordered lots of small plates of delicacies to share among us on a big lazy susan. With the delicacies came a large bowl of white rice. One of our friends was infamously known for never eating his rice, only holding the bowl while feasting on the delicacies. Frugal he may have been, but I also think he rightfully understood that the rice was the filler and not the food.

In the low-fat diet movement of the last part of the 20th century, companies removed fat from their products, replacing it with sugars that made the products more palatable and, frankly, addicting. The industry marketed these reduced-fat or nonfat foods as "healthy" alternatives and may well be directly or indirectly responsible for epidemic levels of obesity and diabetes. The reduced-fat trend was based, at least in part, on calorie counting as a gram of fat has twice the caloric count as a gram of carbohydrate. Dr. Robert Lustig, MD, one of the early voices against the quantities of sugar in our diet, lists fifty-six words used to hide sugar in processed foods on his website. (Lustig)

In the documentary *Sugar: The Bitter Truth*, this history along with references to studies presents the engaging history and consequences of this historic shift in the American diet. (UCTV) Also consider viewing the investigative report *Fed-Up*, which prominently features Dr. Lustig. (David)

The Big "Fat" Lie

In the 1980s and '90s, based on the faulty hypothesis of calories in versus calories out, dietary fat was seen as the main culprit behind increasing obesity because a gram of fat has twice the calories as a gram of protein or carbohydrate. Simultaneously, cholesterol became a primary concern because people believed that eating cholesterol would raise cholesterol levels and increase deposits of cholesterol in the bloodstream, thus increasing risk of cardiovascular disease. Dietary fat was cast in the role of the melodramatic villain of the American diet, making us fat and giving us cardiovascular disease. It was a frame job.

Soon the words "fat free" began showing up on packages all over the supermarket, and such products were labeled as "healthy."

There was even an artificial, calorie-free oil that the body could not process, called Olestra or Olean. Mostly used in processed foods like potato chips, this artificial, indigestible fat had some rather unpleasant side effects and seems to have faded into obscurity.

Of course, removing the fat from processed foods made them less palatable, so while the use of fat decreased, the use of sugar, under its myriad of labels, increased. And Americans got even fatter. The incidence of diabetes skyrocketed, with no real reduction in incidence of cardiovascular disease.

In his video "7 Things Your Doctor got WRONG about Fat," Dr. Ken Berry dispels many of the misconceptions about eating fat. He also provides academic references debunking those misconceptions. (Berry, 7 Things)

LDL cholesterol does appear to go up on a low-carb diet. (Ali) If you and your doctor are concerned about LDL cholesterol and your risk of cardiovascular disease, you may wish to focus some attention on the issues of raised triglycerides, which seem to be a better indicator of risk. Of course, discuss this with your doctor, but also do your own research. A surprising meta study (a review of multiple studies), reported that the relationship between LDL levels and mortality is actually the reverse of what we have traditionally thought. (Ravnskov) Not only that, but the risks associated with LDL cholesterol are made worse by the use of polyunsaturated fats, especially when heated, which actually oxidize and become toxic. (Teicholz, 2015)

Freely eating saturated animal fats has been unfairly demonized in our society, but historically we were healthier before the so-called "healthy" fats were produced. Dr. Chris Knobbe, in his presentation "Diseases of Civilization: Are Seed Oil Excesses the Unifying Mechanism?" presents a logical case for the question. He also provides us with the room to reintroduce some carbohydrates in our diet once our bodies have readjusted, as he references certain tribal societies whose diets consist mainly of unprocessed carbohydrates.

A word of caution: gallbladder removal is one of the most common surgeries in the United States. The purpose of the gallbladder is to collect, concentrate, and store bile for the efficient digestion of fat. Without sufficient fat in the diet, the gall bladder can become sluggish and develop conditions that might lead to the organ being removed. The low-fat diet trend of the last thirty years may be directly or indirectly responsible for the number of gall bladder surgeries. If you have had your gallbladder removed, you will need to be more methodical and gradual in increasing fat in your diet. Your liver still makes bile but will need to ramp up production to accommodate increased fat.

Good Fat vs. Bad Fat

In general, seed oils, corn, sunflower, safflower, canola, etc., are oils that are extracted through a chemical process and are rendered in a form that is not ideal for the absorption of nutrients. Indeed, there is evidence that excessive exposure to these oils has some detrimental effects, including inflammation and possible damage to the gut microbiome. These oils, when heated to the degrees needed for frying, have been demonstrated to produce toxins and a sticky, lacquer-like residue in their environment. (Teicholz, 2015) Given the ubiquitous nature of these oils in many processed foods and in nearly all restaurant food, Americans are just naturally exposed to excessive amounts of them.

If you are taking a supplement that comes in the form of a gel-cap, look at the oil used to carry the nutrition. I suggest you do not waste your money on gel-caps with seed oil carriers, especially those derived through chemical processes. If you need the supplement, it might be rendered more accessible if you took the supplement with a meal higher in natural fats or at least with a natural fat supplement like fish oil.

One mitigating factor is if those oils are labeled as expeller extracted, cold-pressed, or extra virgin. Generally, this means that what you are apparently buying is the easy-to-get, not-chemically-extracted version of these oils.

Good vegetable sources of oil are pure extra virgin olive oil and avocado oil. Olive oil has a low-temperature smoke point and is not the best for frying. Avocado oil is better for cooking as it has a higher smoke point and carries no real flavor of its own. (Cooking) It must be mentioned, however, that some providers of these oils have been cutting higher quality oils with cheap seed oils. (Food Revolution) Just be careful to get the good stuff.

Animal fats—preferably from organic, pasture-raised, pasture-finished livestock—are ideal, unless of course you are a vegetarian. Butter, ghee, lard, and beef tallow are good sources of these oils. Bacon fat is merely lard with a bit of smoky flavor, and if you like bacon, saving that fat and using it to prepare veggies might just help you like veggies a bit better. Vegetarians should carefully choose the oils and fats they use. The article mentioned in the previous paragraph provides a list of safe brands and a list of brands to avoid.

Undoubtedly, in the context of animal fats, the question of cholesterol raises fear. Evidence suggests that triglycerides are more indicative of health risks, including cardiovascular disease, than LDL cholesterol, which may well rise on a lower-carbohydrate, high-fat diet. Whether or not consuming cholesterol, such as that found in egg yolks or bacon, actually raises cholesterol is being constantly debated, depending on who funds the study. One thing we do know is that your body needs and manufactures cholesterol. While most doctors will recommend you take a statin drug to lower-your LDL levels, an increasing number of them are beginning to recommend taking a supplement such as CoQ10 to help mitigate the undesirable consequences of the statin drugs. If you are taking a statin drug, you have some research in your future. (Berry, How to Raise)

What About the Food Pyramid?

They now called it "My Plate," but it amounts to the same thing. (Choose) You would be well-advised to forget the pyramid and the plate! If hypnofasters had their own plate, in terms of bulk, most of our diet might come non-starchy vegetables. Then proteins and fats would be next. And a very small amount of fruit and carbohydrates. If we are to consider the percentage of calories consumed, most calories would come from fat and protein with very controlled amounts of fruit, grains, or other carbohydrates.

There are carbohydrates in vegetables, but vegetables also have fiber, and the amount of carbohydrate by volume in non-starchy vegetables is better balanced and is presumably less processed.

Fresh, organic, non-GMO vegetables are best, but if you have to compromise for financial reasons, stick to organic vegetables that cannot be peeled, like lettuce or spinach. Peeling other vegetables will at least reduce your exposure to topical pesticides. Some veggies are so contaminated that washing does not help. (Parrish, Dirty)

Frozen veggies are better than canned, but it is best to avoid the ones that come packaged with a built-in sauce. I rarely if ever steam my veggies in the plastic bag in which they come, no matter what the directions say. Plastic is plastic, and I do not want to eat it.

If you have to buy canned veggies, at least go for organic and read the labels before you buy them to make sure they are as pure and natural as possible.

If you do not like veggies, it is most likely that you do not know how to prepare them well. It is amazing how many people love green bean casserole on Thanksgiving but will not touch a green bean any other time of the year. Now I am absolutely NOT recommending that casserole because of the processed food used to make it. But I am suggesting giving veggies a chance by preparing them in a variety of ways, using healthy, whole-food ingredients.

I have had clients whose veggie preparation skills involve little more than opening a can and heating the contents. Search a little on the internet, and you will find many recipes that are worth trying. Open your mind to the possibility that you actually do like well-prepared vegetables.

Emotional Eating

Another factor is *why* we eat. Sometimes we feel hungry because of emotional triggers. Emotional eating is a response to mostly unconscious associations of eating with situations, conditions, or circumstances that usually have nothing to do with needing food.

I think many people know about eating as compensation for a rough time or as a reward for being good. We even know from where the mentality comes. A baby cries, and a frustrated parent, who knows the diaper is dry, that the baby is just being fussy for some undetectable reason, gives the baby a cookie or a bowl of dry cereal that is full of sugar and carbohydrates. Baby eats and is placated. The crying stops as the baby is distracted by food. The baby learns that when one feels bad, eat carbs.

"If you clean your room, we will go out for ice cream later." There's bribery for you. Do something good, and I'll reward you or pay you off in some way that involves a treat. It is like paying kids to make their beds, but what do they learn from that? Who is going to pay them to make their beds when they grow up? Sure, they learn how to make a bed, but as an adult, they also have the cash to buy a candy bar, a cup of java so full of sugar it might as well be a milkshake, whether they made their bed or not.

I once knew a woman who, though she lived alone, bought cakes from a bakery on a regular basis. It was not anyone's birthday. There was no festive occasion. She just liked cake with buttercream frosting. "What else do I have?" she responded when I asked her why she had a whole cake on a cake stand under a clear glass cloche on her kitchen table. "I come home from work. I am tired. I am alone. I do not feel like cooking, or I make something quick, and I have a piece of cake to look forward to."

I have to admit, I did enjoy the piece of cake she served me, though today I'd probably thank her but content myself with a cup of black coffee that she expertly made in a French press. The point is that the cake was for her either a compensation or reward or even just a form of comfort.

You do not need to compensate for having a bad day. You almost certainly have them, of course, but so does everyone. Neither do you need to reward myself for living your life in a positive way. Take notice when you find yourself rewarding or compensating yourself. Find better ways to do that.

If you need comforting, then you need comforting—not a huge plate of food. Intermittent fasting with an LCHF diet has literally changed my life, as it will yours, if you let it. When I feel I need comforting, I *do* something comforting, not eat something comforting. I might take some time off work. I might take a drive to a different area. Go browse at a regular clothing store now that I can actually fit into the clothes they sell. I might work on a hobby or craft. I might watch a video or putter around in my garden. I might meet a friend for coffee or, if no one is available, go myself and people-watch.

Most of us are already familiar with that kind of emotional eating, but I am a hypnotist. I am trained to know the power that language has on the unconscious mind. Let me introduce you to something a little deeper in the unconscious.

Cravings

We have all experienced cravings in one form or another. Some people believe they crave certain foods because their body needs the nutrients those foods contain. It would be wonderful if that were true. But how does one explain craving a donut? There is nothing nutritional in a donut. I suppose it could be attributable to sugar addiction. There are times when we will crave something sweet. But why, then, might a craving be so specific? Unless there is some chemical dependency, cravings are triggered by a mental or emotional association.

If you think about it, you will notice that a craving for a particular food is almost always an "away from" motivation that masquerades as a "toward" motivation. I think I want a donut, but what I really want is to not think about or avoid something unpleasant. Perhaps my boss just gave me another task. Perhaps I had a difficult conversation with my spouse. Perhaps I am feeling stressed, depressed, or fatigued.

Intellectually we understand that the donut does not really provide anything beyond a momentary distraction and a fleeting sugar high, but those temporary benefits seem to outweigh the looming issue, whatever it may be.

When you find yourself experiencing cravings, instead of seeking the object of your urge, stop and take a look at what you are experiencing or thinking. What caused the craving? If you address the issue, the craving will disappear. Do this often enough, and you will actually rewire your brain to break the connection between the triggering issue and the craving.

If you experience persistent cravings or have difficulty identifying the issue behind them, you should address the topic with your hypnotist. To find a hypnotist trained in The Hypnofasting Program, visit our website, www.hypnofastingprogram.com.

Your Internal Monologue

We have already explored the difference between being hungry and feeling hungry. When we say we are hungry, we are, in very subtle ways, identifying with that feeling. It very gently becomes part of our identity rather than just describing a temporary feeling. If I declare that I *am* hungry, it is like subtly saying something about me, as a person. But if I say I *feel* hungry, I am merely describing a temporary condition.

It may just be a problem in English. In Spanish, for example, there is no equivalent for I am hungry. The Spanish phrase is "Tengo hambre." or "I have hunger." Having hunger says nothing about me or my value as a person. True, both the English and Spanish phrases communicate the same concept—one feels hungry—but unconsciously, they are not the same thing. Any bilingual person knows that thoughts and concepts change when speaking a different language. There are words, phrases, and even concepts that cannot be translated with any degree of accuracy because the context is cultural, not merely linguistic. Many people who learn a second language as an adult spend the rest of their lives trying to translate between the two languages because the culture is missing. One has to immerse oneself in the culture to gain any understanding at all.

You see, most people live their lives with a kind of running monologue or narration in their minds. Our thoughts are expressed in language. And language affects the brain.

The internal monologue did not always exist. When we were babies, we experienced things without the use of language because there were no words in our heads to describe things. About the closest we come to experiencing something as we did when we were infants is when something leaves us speechless. Still, we have words for that experience: awestruck, gobsmacked, astonished, or astounded, or even good old speechless.

In English, mindless emotional eating is often associated with an "I am…" phrase or thought. When I am working with an emotional eater, I always try to get them to identify their "I am" statements. Because we have learned to define our experiences using language. If our native language is English, we have built in an autosuggestion mechanism, a kind of self-hypnosis. We are absolutely barraged with constantly reinforced "I am" statements and thoughts that settle in our unconscious minds, becoming part of our identity rather than merely describing what is most often a temporary condition.

I am sad. I am fat. I am depressed. I am confused. I am lonely. I am a victim. I am pathetic. I am stupid. I am unpopular.

Of course, positive statements work as well. I am happy. I am attractive. I am comfortable. I am popular. I am normal. I am exceptional. I am terrific. I am great.

Balancing the negative and positive "I am" statements comes down to sheer numbers, and therein we find our redemption.

Once we identify our negative "I am" thoughts, we can call them out, examine them, change them, reverse them. This is the whole idea behind affirmations. We consciously try to monitor and adjust the balance of our "I am" thoughts so that we can effectively change our experience.

If you are an emotional eater, try to identify the "I am" thoughts or statements that result in emotional eating, whether for compensation or reward, or even avoidance (eating to distract yourself from attending to something daunting or unpleasant). This process can be difficult and will require some soul searching as these patterns are often deeply seated in the unconscious mind. Often, emotional eaters have difficulty working through a veritable montage of them.

Your hypnotist should be able to help you do this. We use a lot of techniques to isolate and define them. Merely defining them is occasionally enough. When we understand patterns of thought that were created when we were little, our adult understanding can see through that process. Most often, however, we need to process the change through other hypnotic techniques and occasionally, really rarely, a person might need to address the issue with a mental health therapist or counselor. Your hypnotist should be able to know if that is the case and might have a referral for you.

If you identify these "I am" thoughts on your own, you can attempt to change them consciously. First rephrase them. Convert the declaration of being to a description of a temporary feeling or emotion. Consciously reword the phrase from "I am" to "I feel."

Every time the thought happens or the urge to inexplicably eat presents itself, reinforce the change. Then develop a statement about yourself, a kind of affirmation, that counteracts the force of the old pattern. Like the woman who came home tired to a lonely house to eat cake, consider creating a statement like this: "I have had a busy day and now can rest."

When I started this process, I composed a rather long phrase that countered my feelings of hunger and the compulsion to snack. I repeated it to myself when I knew I did not need to eat. (I had already planned what and when I would eat again.) "My body is adjusting and healing itself at this very moment. My cells are relearning insulin sensitivity, and my liver is using up what it has stored." This mantra or affirmation helped me bolster my ability to stick with my plan.

Hunger comes in waves. It will pass. We need to learn that feeling hungry does not mean we *need* to eat.

Extending Your Fast

From your Stage One fasting journal, consider the times of your natural fast—that is, the time between your final bite yesterday and your first bite today. You should have at least a week of numbers. Let's get an average of those numbers. Add up all the numbers and divide by the number of fasts you have tracked. The answer is your average natural fast. For some, it may be as few as six or eight hours. For others, it may be twelve or fourteen.

Your average natural fast is now your minimum fast and, in this stage, we will make every attempt to increase that number by two hours every day.

Example: John tracked his natural fasts over the last seven days. Those fasts were ten, nine, nine, eight, eleven, eight, and nine. Add up the numbers and you get sixty-four. Divide sixty-four by seven, and his natural fast was a little longer than nine hours. Nine hours is now John's minimum fast. When he swallows his last bite today, he looks at the clock. If it is 8:30 p.m., John understands that his next bite of food should not take place for nine hours, until after 5:30 a.m.

But wait…we are *extending* the fast. We want to broaden the natural fast by two hours. So really, John's next bite should not happen until after 7:30 a.m. John may eat after 5:30, but he should not eat until after 7:30 a.m.

Whether John chooses to finish eating earlier the day before or start eating later the next day, his goal for this stage is to obtain an average natural fast of eleven hours. He will stay in this stage until that happens. *Whatever your natural fast, extend it by two hours.*

When scheduling your fasts, tell yourself that you can or should eat after (not at) your corresponding times. If you plant the idea in your mind that you will eat at a specific time, I can almost guarantee you will be ravenous at that time. But if you phrase the goal as eating after that time, you will have less urgency to eat.

It is also really important to plan what you will eat to *break* your fast. (That's where the word breakfast comes from. But it can happen anytime, not just in the morning.) You do not want to reach for the nearest thing. If you plan, you will break your fast with good food that you will look forward to eating. You will break your fast with food that you will be able to eat more mindfully. You will be less likely to overeat when you break your fast.

Cutting the Carbs

Remember those mental images of your portions? Here is where they come in handy. You knew I was going to get there, did you not? This step does not have to be complicated, and if you are like most of us and your diet has virtually centered around carbs, the thought of cutting them out entirely might be quite scary. After all, what the heck are you going to eat?

Let's keep it simple for now. Just remove half of them from your plate. If you are eating a hamburger, eat it with a knife and fork and forget the top of the bun. If that burger comes with fries, are there other options? If not, just eat half of them. When you take your portions, be aware of the amount you would normally take and just help yourself to half.

When making entries into your food journal, talk about the cuts you have made and how you feel about those changes. You see, if you feel terribly restricted, you may need to take things slowly until your motivation builds. When I started out, I cut my carbs in half, and in a week or so, I realized that I did not have to eat many of them at all. I had other choices. Over time, I gradually eliminated quite a few carbs entirely.

Remember that to make sustainable change, we have to do it in a way that does not feel overly restrictive. We have to allow for the possibility of a larger or different change later. Now, when I order a hamburger, I do not even want the bun. I do not miss it at all. I ask them to leave it off. If they forget, it just means that I leave it on the plate. I do not want to eat it. If my burger comes with fries, and I cannot exchange the fries for something else, someone at the table is always, and I mean always, willing to eat my fries.

You will not have to eliminate all carbohydrates for the rest of your life. We want our bodies to heal. We want a newer, lower carbohydrate normal, and we want our bodies to adjust, requiring a more appropriate insulin response. There will come a time when you may gradually add back in some chosen carbohydrates. You will have some wiggle room. But, honestly, you will not want to wiggle as much as you think you would.

Joseph A. Onesta

Chapter 6
Stage Three

The Most Important Meal?

Breakfast is the most important meal of the day, right? The truthful answer is simple. No, not if you understand breakfast to be an early morning meal. In fact, it is fairly likely that breakfast being the "most important meal" was just an advertising ploy to sell boxed cereal.

Traditional American breakfasts are usually full of carbohydrates, which are quickly digested and cause a spike in blood sugar with a rapid insulin response, resulting in feelings of hunger in a noticeably short time. If you have trouble making it to lunch even after a big breakfast, you know what I am talking about. One client reported to me that when he ate pancakes, he felt overly full and could hardly finish his plate, but within an hour or so, he would be looking for a snack.

Redefine breakfast as a meal that breaks your natural fast. That meal can come anytime. It is entirely an artificial construct to think that breakfast happens in the morning hours. Who cares if the local diner says breakfast is served before 11 a.m.? You can break your fast anytime you like.

Naming meals as breakfast, lunch, or dinner only means when you have eaten one, you have not eaten the others, and, psychologically, you expect to eat again. Mentally, you have not finished eating until after dinner.

I hardly think of our cave-dwelling ancestors arguing over whether the meal they were eating was technically breakfast, lunch, or brunch, especially since they might not eat again for quite some time. If I have "lunch" at 3 p.m., do I have to have dinner even if I am not hungry? If I eat bacon and eggs at 6 p.m., is it breakfast or dinner? Who cares? The whole idea that we need three square meals a day is simply a fallacy.

From now on, we decide when and what we will eat. And we will eat it consciously. Mindfully.

The first meal I eat after a fast is my break-fast meal, and I can have any kind of food that is not laden with carbohydrates. Forget pancakes, oatmeal, toast, bread, croissants, cereals, or any kind of grain or sugar-based foods. If you have to eat that stuff, eat it at some other time. They are not appropriate foods for breaking a fast.

Protein and fat are better macronutrient choices for breaking a fast. Protein digests slowly, and fat lends itself to a feeling of satiety for a longer period of time. Bacon and eggs are a good traditional choice. A hearty soup or stew made with bone broth, meat, and vegetables is a great way to break a fast. If you are vegetarian or vegan, an organic tofu scramble with some sauteed kale, spinach, or chard would be quite nice.

Do Calories Count?

We do not count calories to lose weight. Anyone who has yo-yo dieted knows that regaining lost weight is cake walk...pun intended.

Anyway, not all calories are processed in the same way. We do not count calories, but they still count...in a way.

Your body is used to consuming a certain number of calories. A severely reduced calorie diet will cause you to lose weight, but your brain-body naturally assumes the restriction in calories is temporary and that the reduction in weight is also meant to be temporary. Think of excess fat as your body's emergency fund, a way of saving up for a rainy day. The diet comes, and your body assumes it is raining. When you have achieved your target weight, it is the most natural thing in the world to want to get back to normal. You feel great, attractive, even sexy, and that piece of pie is a well-deserved treat, right?

Wrong. You have starved your body of nutrients, and it has begun rationing energy. If you have ever had to rely on your savings during a period of unemployment, you probably became very frugal with your money. Your body does the same thing with its fuel when you sustain a reduced calorie diet. It gets frugal. Your body has, in a way, learned to function on far fewer calories. Any increase in caloric intake consequently is used to replenish your body's depleted savings. Let me make that clear. When you start eating a normal diet again, your body just uses the caloric increase to make fat.

In The Hypnofasting Program, we are not just losing weight or getting our blood sugar under control so then we can go back to doing what we were doing before. We do not want to go back to that normal. We did not like that normal. We want a new normal.

We do not count calories to lose weight because restricting our calories causes frugality to kick in. Granted, we may have had an artificially high caloric intake, and we may discover that we really do not need to eat that much. But that comes in a far later stage of The Hypnofasting Program process. Won't it be lovely to eat until you are satisfied while being completely in control of your cravings?

Until then, we remain aware of what we are eating to establish and maintain a healthy metabolism. That means we do not intentionally reduce our caloric intake. We do not go into starvation mode. Our bodies get and have enough nutrition to not only survive, but thrive.

Our bodies have protocols for using nutrients. Our bodies know what to do with carbohydrates, proteins, and fats, and our bodies do different things with those nutrients. Based on our weight and/or our insulin resistance, we have determined that we have a surplus of glucose in our bodies. We therefore avoid overstuffing our bodies with carbohydrates and sugar so that our bodies can use the reserves, while we provide sufficient protein and fat to maintain our metabolism and improve our health.

Do not put yourself on a restricted calorie diet. If you are not sure you are eating enough, eat until you are full then stop. If you do not know what it is like to feel full, then set a time limit. If you can plan to eat after a certain hour, you can plan to stop eating after a reasonable time has passed. If you sit down to eat at noon, you can tell yourself you are finished eating at 12:30, for example. At 12:30, get up from the table and don't eat again until the next planned meal.

For more detailed explanations about calories, consider the following three YouTube videos: "The Calorie Deception," by Dr. Jason Fung, (Fung, The Calorie) "Berry, Why Calories Do Not Count" (Berry, Why Calories) and "Counting Calories is Stupid" (Berry, Counting).

If you are maintaining a vegetarian or vegan lifestyle, I am afraid you may still need to think about calories but not count them as in a reduced calorie diet. Because vegetarian or vegan sources of protein are also often sources of carbohydrates, attempting to maintain protein levels while cutting carbohydrates can be a challenge. Cutting carbs may also mean cutting some proteins. Vegetarians and vegans may find it necessary to determine what percentage of their calories or portions of food come from protein and carbohydrates, and adjust accordingly.

Adjusting to Changes

Often when I am working with clients, they express reservations about their ability to accept some of the changes we will make. One client dubbed herself the "Carbohydrate Queen" and resisted cutting her consumption of many carbohydrates. She was using her self-imposed label to justify her resistance to the kinds of changes we needed. "I know myself," she asserted.

We worked on this notion in hypnosis, and she came to realize that she resisted the changes because, in the back of her mind, she thought that eventually she could never have a carbohydrate again. This idea was certainly her own creation. Indeed, there will be changes that we live out for the rest of our lives, but eliminating all carbohydrates completely forever was never part of the program. The very idea is not only the antithesis of motivation; that is ridiculous.

The Hypnofasting Program is not about never having cake, bread, or pasta again. It is about being in touch with your body, giving it what it needs to heal, recover, and change. Once you have established your new normal, you will know if and how much cake, bread, or pasta is good for you.

Remember, our changes are incremental. We are going from stage to stage, and while doing that, we are making up for lost ground. The Hypnofasting Program provides a time for recovery and rejuvenation. We are working up to a goal, but when we reach it, there will be a period of stabilization, followed by a kind of warm-down that settles into your new normal.

I give you this information like a mountain guide who tells you what it is like at the summit, but then says something like, "You cannot know what it is really like until you get there."

The Eating Window

As we continue to increase the number of fasting hours, the hours remaining in the day constitute our eating window. This window is important to us because it is our opportunity to convince our bodies that everything is all right. We are not starving, and there is no need to go into emergency energy conservation mode.

It is important that we eat well during our eating window. That does not mean eating untold quantities of anything that happens to be available. It does not mean snacking the whole time. It does not mean "treating" ourselves to things we are supposed to be cutting down. Eating well means eating good, fresh, whole, nutritious food that will deliver the nutrients and energy we need without triggering too much insulin production.

Planning what you will eat is possibly the best way of avoiding scarfing up whatever happens to be handy. It is also the best way to make sure we are eating food that is nutritious and delicious.

If you are out when your eating window is open, either plan what you will buy and make sure you can get it or pack your food and take it with you. Invariably, at some point in your journey, something unexpected may happen, and you find yourself with nothing worth eating.

The very concept of there being food that is not worth eating is probably new to most people, but it is one of the hallmarks of a hypnofaster. Something worth eating is something that will not only quell our feeling of hunger but will nourish our bodies and help our systems to continue their healing and restoration processes. Anything that goes counter to those purposes is not worth eating.

It is not about what you can and cannot have. But when you have internalized what is worth eating, you will find it easier and more satisfying to simply not eat rather than consuming something not worth eating.

Increasing your consumption of truly healthy fats will do three things. First, you will more easily maintain a normal, more sustainable, caloric intake. Second, because of the way fat is digested, you will naturally experience fewer feelings of hunger and the feeling of satiety will last longer. Third, you will be allowing your body to access and use fat as a fuel in an appropriate way.

Our ultimate goal in extending the natural fast is to find the eating window that causes us to use up the nutrients we consume and draw on our stores of fat. Later, when there are not huge quantities of fat that need using up, we adjust a little more and settle into our new normal.

Some people think that as their eating window narrows, they still have to consume three meals. You do not. Just go to two full meals with no snacking in between.

"Microdosing" Sugar

Remember how the processed food industry replaced fat with sugar in the '80s and the '90s when the phrase "fat free" became a big selling point? The food industry used sugar in various forms as a flavor enhancer, even in products that are not meant to be sweet, like soup. As our dependence on manufactured food increased, the result was that people consumed tiny amounts of sugar, what I call a "microdose," in nearly all their food.

Sugar under any of its names, according to Lustig, is a "chronic dose dependent hepatotoxin." Those big words mean that sugar poisons your liver, and the more you eat of it, the more toxic it is. In other words, it all adds up—even in tiny amounts over a long period of time.

When we add in the sugar found in foods that are supposed to be sweet, the quantity of sugar consumed by the average American in a year is staggering. I have seen estimates ranging from 62 to 152 pounds per year. When a single eight-ounce, soft drink contains more than eight teaspoons of sugar, these numbers are not difficult to believe.

Sugar gave the food industry two key advantages. First, it is cheap, especially since not all sugar is actually sugar. Remember: there's cane sugar, but there is also beet sugar, high fructose corn syrup, and then all those other names for sugar. (Lustig) They are dirt cheap compared to other ingredients.

Cheap sugars have a secondary and very profitable side effect; sugar is addictive. (Avena)

Maps of the brains of people who have ingested sugar virtually match those who have been given cocaine. (Nunes) Lab animals, when given a choice between sugary water and cocaine, choose the sweet drink hands down. (Devoskin)

So, not only did the food industry gain a cheap, flavor-enhancing ingredient, it was able to introduce a substance that naturally and legally prompted people to crave and buy more of it.

Now take a few moments to get a few of these products from your kitchen:

- Ketchup
- Canned soup
- Bottled salad dressing
- Boxed cereal
- Mayonnaise
- Any frozen meal

Read the list of ingredients and look for two things. How many times in different forms does sugar appear on the list? And how early in the list does the first one appear?

The earlier in the list the item appears, the higher percentage of that ingredient is in the product. On many products, you may well find sugar to be among the first three ingredients. It may even appear several more times again on the list. Add it all up, and even a tablespoon of ketchup might constitute a fix.

Add to this the understanding that ingredients that add carbohydrates are just another form that the body sees as sugar, things like potato or cornstarch, any grain, any form of fruit or juice.

Sugar is not benign, and the American diet is full of sugar and carbohydrates. This is arguably and scientifically the source of most obesity and the epidemic of type 2 diabetes.

Sugar has also been demonstrated to play a role in cancer progression, digestive disorders like IBS and Crohn's disease, mood disorders, chronic fatigue, and fibromyalgia.

Sucrose and Fructose

Regular granulated sugar is about 50% sucrose and about 50% fructose. This is important to us for one main reason. Sucrose can be processed by virtually every cell in the body. If we consume a reduced amount of carbohydrates and are sufficiently active (we will talk about activity later), it is possible for our bodies to need and use the glucose in our blood stream straight away.

Remember it is *excess* glucose that is stored in the liver. If the body needs glucose and there isn't any available, the liver will make it out of fat. At first, the process is called gluconeogenesis—that is, making glucose from fat. Later, your liver may choose to produce ketones, another fuel your body thrives on, but that comes much later.

Fructose, on the other hand, can only be processed in the liver. When the food industry says that high-fructose corn syrup is just another form of sugar, it is true, but that is not the whole story. Every drop, grain, or atom of fructose is sent straight to the liver. The less fructose we consume, the less our liver is distracted by having to process it. When we consume sugar or fructose in any form, including fresh fruit, our liver has to work.

In order to lose weight and control type 2 diabetes, we want our fatigued livers to heal and begin to access stored fat energy. With reduced need for insulin, our bodies are not attempting to find places to store the excess. Our sensitivity to insulin increases.

Extending Your Fast—Again!

In this stage, extend your daily fast another two hours. If you remember John from the last stage, he is now going from eleven hours to thirteen. We want to accomplish two things. We want you to be more comfortable with not eating. That fact becomes a sign that your brain-body is adjusting to intentional or mindful eating. Also, we want to establish the level of fasting that will have the most positive effect on your progress.

While it is an individual process, most of us will work our way up to a regular fast of sixteen to eighteen hours every day, leaving a eating window of six to eight hours with very occasional shorter periods of fasting and intermittent longer ones. Though you may already be there, the goal of sixteen to eighteen hours of normal fasting is one we will achieve in Stage Four. If you are already there, that is, your normal fast is at least sixteen hours, just keep steady. Perhaps push it to eighteen hours once or twice.

Cutting Even More Carbs

Try cutting them in half again and perhaps eliminating some altogether. You may choose to learn some new recipes for keto replacements for things like bread or crackers. (YouTube is chock full of keto cooks.) There may be a lot of disappointment there, but for those who cannot imagine a bun-less burger or hotdog, these options can help you get through. Early on I tried several versions of keto bread, and they were OK...but just OK. I also tried several recipes for keto noodles, none to my satisfaction.

Chapter 7
Stage Four

Staying Hydrated

Often, when we think we feel hungry, we are really thirsty. Humans can go an exceptionally long time without food, but without water we might live only three or four days. It is important for you to keep hydrated, not only because it helps you avoid feeling hungry, but because dehydration can be a real problem. Some of the side-effects people experience often attribute to fasting, such as light-headedness, dizziness, headache, drowsiness, or a lack of energy, are really side effects of dehydration. A good, tall glass of water should do the trick.

There are many things you can drink during a fast that will not interrupt your progress, and you can drink as much as you want. Just remember that there should be no sugar, no carbohydrates, and no artificial sweeteners in the beverage.

Purified or filtered water is the best, and if you need flavor, squeeze in a wedge of lemon or lime and/or a splash of raw apple cider vinegar. That bit of juice will not make much difference, and it adds flavor. If you miss the fizz of soda pop, consider seltzer water instead of filtered water.

You can drink coffee or tea. Black is best, but if you need to augment it, use heavy cream or a bit of coconut oil. These will cause the least interruption of your fast. You can add spices, just not sugar. Avoid artificial creamers and sweeteners because of their chemical composition. A cup of hot water with a squeeze of lemon or apple cider vinegar makes for a change. Herbal teas can taste a bit sweet and help if you are sensitive to caffeine. Don't forget that both coffee and tea can be quite refreshing iced as well as hot.

Part of hydration is consuming sufficient salt. Like fat, salt has been vilified in our society, and the concepts behind reducing salt in the diet have questionable provenance. I am convinced that the recommendations to restrict salt are meant to compensate for the copious amounts of salt in processed or manufactured foods. Since hypnofasters are avoiding those foods, we may need to invest in some healthy sea or deep-mine salt that also contributes trace minerals to our diet. If you are eating well, that is, eating good whole foods, there is no need to fear adding salt to your food. (Berry, Is Salt)

Naturally, you might be afraid of adding salt to your diet because you may be concerned about your blood pressure. High blood pressure is indeed something to be concerned about, but let's not blame salt. Your body needs salt. Take a few moments to learn from Dr. Berry on how to lower your blood pressure naturally. (Berry, Lower)

Circadian Rhythms

When we think about what is normal for us, we must understand that we have an internal timing mechanism called our "circadian rhythm." This natural cycle comes with some universal presets that, over time, we override or change.

For example, one universal preset is that darkness generally signals time to sleep, but there are people who consider themselves night owls. They seem to get their energy as the sun goes down. Virtually everyone likes things that are sweet. It is theorized that this desire for sweet things evolved over epochs to cause us to store energy for lean times. Of course, for most of us in the western world, lean times rarely come.

These preset alerts can be changed by consistent habit. If you normally eat a bowl of sugary cereal for breakfast, bacon and eggs might not satisfy you because you find yourself craving sugar. Of course, if you replace the sugary cereal with bacon and eggs over a long enough period of time, the sugar cravings will disappear, and you will be more than satisfied with bacon and eggs.

Additionally, if you were a breakfast eater and have been extending your natural fast during the morning hours, you probably had a little trouble getting through the morning without thinking about food. That will change.

Any sustained pattern in life can reset the alerts on your circadian clock. The process is akin to coping with jet lag when a person eventually grows accustomed to a new time zone. Until we have reached our goals, we want to be careful about establishing patterns too soon. Even the sixteen- to eighteen-hour natural fast needs to be shaken up once in a while so that the brain-body does not assume it is a new normal and settle into a new pattern too soon.

If you have dieted before, you have probably experienced a plateau, meaning that the changes just stopped. You were stuck. You were not losing any more weight. A plateau means the brain body is assuming a new normal. Establishing patterns, even on The Hypnofasting Program, can bring about a plateau. If you find yourself getting completely comfortable in a pattern of behavior, shake it up, change it.

If you experience a kind of holding pattern at any point during this program, we can shake things up in several ways. We might schedule in an extended fast. We might choose to eat more or less for a time. We might choose to eat something different. We might change our routine or eat at different times. Making the first meal of the day the largest instead of waiting for dinner might be a sufficient change. Discuss other options with your hypnotherapist.

The only thing that should be absolutely regular is your sleep. If you are working with a hypnotist, he or she should have asked you how well you sleep. While sleep behaviors are not really part of The Hypnofasting Program, they are critical for your health.

Sleep deprivation causes stress, and stress releases cortisol, which makes it difficult to lose weight. Try going to bed at the same time each night and getting out of bed the same time each morning. This pattern will begin to reset that circadian rhythm. The need for eight to ten hours of sleep a night, deep enough to include both rapid eye movement (REM) and non-REM sleep, is optimal. (Walker)

Sometimes there are physiological conditions that disrupt sleep. Sleep apnea (when a person stops breathing momentarily during sleep) or the urgent need to urinate in the middle of the night interrupts the natural patterns. Our overuse of LED lights and electronic devices may inhibit the production of melatonin, which is our body's natural mechanism for signaling sleepiness. Tension, stress, and mounting anxiety are often psychological causes for disrupted sleep patterns.

If you are genuinely having trouble with your sleep, your hypnotherapist should be able to help you. Most of us have helped many clients sleep better.

The Dawn Phenomenon

One circadian pattern many diabetics notice is called the "Dawn Phenomenon." In preparation for waking up, the body begins to increase levels of certain hormones, and this causes an increase in blood sugar. In many who are insulin resistant, the increase in blood glucose levels is more marked.

When I first noticed this, I became alarmed. I thought my body was going crazy because my blood sugar levels went up even though I had fasted. But with a bit of research I learned that the rise in blood glucose was a natural thing. If I used my body and moved my muscles during that period of elevated blood glucose, I had the opportunity to actually further my progress by *using* the energy available to me rather than waiting for insulin to do the balancing act for me. It seemed logical to me that if there was glucose in the blood, activity might just encourage my cells to be less insulin resistant. Using energy stored in cells through activity naturally makes them more receptive to the delivery of more energy by getting it out of the blood.

It is best to simply test your blood glucose levels just before your first meal, rather than when you wake up. If I test my blood before my first meal, and I notice the levels are still a little high, I postpone eating and do something physical. I might stretch, go out into my garden, putter around in my basement, clean the kitchen, cut the grass, or take a long walk. If I do not have time for that sort of thing, I just go about my business not eating and checking my blood glucose every couple of hours.

I never take a fasting lab blood test before 10 a.m. Back in the day when fasting was a chore, I went to the lab at 6 a.m. when it opened, so I could eat after. Now, eating is not so urgent, my readings are lower, and I feel better about them. Of course, my A1c is what the doctor mostly cares about, so I'm not fooling anybody about my blood sugar levels. My A1c has been consistently below prediabetic levels for more than a year.

Blood Glucose Alert!

If you are not taking medications for diabetes, you are unlikely to ever have to deal with low blood sugar levels. You might feel hungry. You might feel tired and cranky, and you might even feel a little cloudy from time to time, but your body has a natural way of balancing things out.

The important thing to know is that if you are curled up on your bed, clutching your gut in wrenching hunger, eat something: a few nuts or olives, a bit of cheese, a hard-boiled egg. The Hypnofasting Program is designed to gradually help you move from one stage to the next.

However, if you are taking medications for type 2 diabetes, the longer you fast without adjusting your medications, the more low-blood sugar risk you face.

Monitor your blood sugar levels aggressively. I tested my sugar levels eight or nine times a day because everything was changing and low blood sugar is nasty. I would use a different finger each time, but ouch!

It is wonderful to see levels that are normal. I relished those normal levels when I experienced them, but it soon became obvious that if I continued my medications at the prescribed level, and I continued to cut carbs and increase my fasts, I might soon experience low blood sugar...and I did. If you are not certain about the symptoms of low blood sugar, I urge you to educate yourself. (Symptoms)

If you have not already done so, please contact your physician to explain your process and the amount you are testing your blood. If your blood glucose levels are responding well, your doctor will give you instructions for reducing your medications. It may be as simple as buying a pill cutter. But it may also mean a change in medications. This process is something your doctor should prescribe and monitor.

Of course, when I cut down my medications, my levels increased slightly, but they leveled off fairly quickly. That, in my mind, signaled not only more appropriate insulin levels, but that my cells were becoming more sensitive to the insulin I was manufacturing. There is a lab test for the doctor to measure your insulin resistance called the "Homeostatic Insulin Resistance Test." I admit I have never had the test performed as I was consistently satisfied with my blood sugar monitoring results.

Weeding out the Microdoses of Sugar

Now is the time to start eliminating, as much as possible, the microdoses of sugar. Start at the level at which you are comfortable and then challenge yourself bit by bit.

Some people who have the available finances can purge their cupboards of the processed food that contains hidden sugars and filler carbohydrates and replace them with better versions, if better versions exist. You can find ketchup, mayonnaise, and cocktail sauce without added sugars. They may be pricey, but they are available. You might consider just making your own. You may find your homemade version is better than the one you buy.

Some things you will simply eliminate entirely. I do not use ketchup anymore. I tried some expensive brands of ketchup that had no added sugar, and frankly, ketchup was not worth that kind of money. I twice tried to make my own but was frustrated by my inability to get the seasoning right.

When I examined my own use of ketchup, I realized that it only served to make certain foods, like french fries, more palatable. I do not eat many french fries anymore, as a rule. I still use condiments, just not ketchup. Burgers, hot dogs, and the occasional fry from my husband's plate get a dip in mustard...divine. Most mustards do not have added sugars, and I like the taste.

So, I buy the regular ketchup for my husband, who cannot seem to live without it, and who is not diabetic. Anyway, I am the family cook, and since there are very few microdoses of sugar in our pantry, he can have his ketchup.

Brain-Body Communication

Everything we experience is a product of a conversation between the brain and the body. The brain can cause the body to react. Physical, mental, or emotional experiences are integrally related to processes in the brain. Our hearts race, for example, when we are afraid whether that fear is reasonable or not.

The mechanical processes of the brain are complex, but we can simplify them for our purposes. Your brain and your body are in communication all the time.

Consider this scene. You are invited to a picnic or barbecue. As you get close to the event, you start thinking about the fun you will have and the variety of food you will eat. Uncle Frank's famous ribs with his homemade secret sauce. Aunt Millie's equally famous rhubarb pie. Whether you are focused on the ribs or the pie or both, you likely begin feeling hungry just thinking about it. Even the unpleasant smell of the charcoal grill being lit with lighter fluid might make you salivate.

At the prospect of that food, often linked to your expected enjoyment, your body reacts further by generating increased digestive fluids. Your heart rate may actually shift a bit. And, believe it or not, your body will begin to produce insulin in response to the expectation of food to come.

I am convinced that frisbees, volleyball, and gossip are just fun ways of distracting us until the food is ready. I do not need to mention, of course, the pretzels, chips, and the coolers full of beer and soda pop that tide picnickers over in anticipation.

In normal, healthy individuals, there are checks and balances that monitor the system and compensate for inaccurate expectations. But in insulin-resistant folks, the system has glitches. An insulin-resistant body has trouble making those automatic adjustments.

When it is discovered that Aunt Millie dropped the pie as she was leaving the house that morning or Uncle Frank says the ribs will not be ready for several hours, a healthy body simply adjusts. Those functions slow or stop. But if your body is insulin resistant, you may be less able to cope with such changes. Aunt Millie suddenly becomes a clumsy old bitty and Uncle Frank should have known better than to buy the discount charcoal.

You feel disappointment, even irritability, despite the fact that Aunt Millie and Uncle Frank have expressed their regrets. An insulin-resistant person might actually encounter unexpected emotions that result in copious amounts of pretzels, chips, and beer or soda being irrationally consumed.

The process by which your pancreas secretes more insulin in anticipation of food is called the "cephalic insulin response." The word cephalic indicates that the cause of the response is mental, not physical. Sucking on a hard candy naturally causes more saliva. As a boy scout, I learned that sucking on a button when no water was available would quell my thirst, at least for a while. That response is physical.

If I ask you to close your eyes and take you through guided imagery mimicking giving you a lemon-drop candy and have you place it in your mouth, you may well notice a saliva increase, even a slight pucker expecting the sour taste. Because of your memory of the flavor, you may actually taste the lemon drop. That is a cephalic response.

Given that information, it should not surprise you to know that your pancreas may well begin secreting insulin to counter the expected influx of sugar in the lemon drop, even if it is an imaginary one.

This is why eating needs to become more conscious, especially for those of us in recovery from some form or degree of insulin resistance. When we learn to quell cephalic, irrational hunger and eat consciously or mindfully, we teach our brain-body to distrust irrational feelings of hunger and begin to react more sensitively to the intentional nature of eating.

Imagine if your body began insulin secretion only when you actually sat down to a meal.

Artificial and Nonnutritive Sweeteners

There are many good reasons to avoid artificial sweeteners. (Strawbridge) Not all artificial sweeteners are created equal. In addition to artificial sweetener effects on blood sugar and body weight, researchers have examined the relationship between nonnutritive (artificial) sweeteners and oral health, eating behaviors, mood and brain function, and risks for cancer, cardiovascular disease, and kidney disease. (Shmerling)

In terms of The Hypnofasting Program, the cephalic insulin response explains one important reason why artificial sweeteners are counterproductive. After all, we want to require less, not more, insulin.

When you eat something sweet, your tongue only knows that it is sweet and that taste usually means sugar is coming into the body. Sensing sweet, your tongue sends a message to your brain. "Hey, head's up. We got sugar on the way!"

Your brain then relays the message to your stomach, your pancreas, and your liver, all of which respond in kind. Your stomach gets ready for digestion. Your pancreas starts to secrete insulin and your liver gets ready for more storage, which also means it may well stop gluconeogenesis (converting glycogen or even fat into glucose).

In other words, your fast has ended, even though you may have consumed nothing more than a glass of chemicals from a diet soda pop, or you may even just be chewing some sugar-free gum.

What do you do if an expected guest does not show up? You call.

What do you imagine happens when the stomach does not get the sugar it expects? It calls. Imagine that response multiplied in the insulin-resistant person.

Your stomach sends a message to your brain, which goes something like this. "Hey! What happened? Where's the sugar you promised?"

Your brain then does not know what happened even though intellectually you do. So the brain begins to send all sorts of signals in order to get the sugar it thought it was going to get when your taste buds registered something sweet. Immediately, you start to crave sweets and/or carbohydrates, like chips, or bread, which, as you know, merely turn to glucose in your system. While you enjoyed the sweet taste of the soda pop, your body was confused and responded accordingly.

The cephalic insulin response varies in different people, but whether the sweetener is artificial or is a natural nonnutritive sweetener, like pure Stevia, the potential for insulin secretion can be the same.

Though to my knowledge, unsubstantiated, the same brain-body confusion may happen when we consume food that is not really food but a chemical concoction that merely resembles food. Chemically laden manufactured foods (including forms of vitamin "enrichments" that the body cannot absorb and oils that the body does not recognize as legitimate, healthy, nutrition-carrying fat) may cause the brain-body to react in unexpected ways. (Major players are seed and vegetable oils that must be chemically extracted, margarine, vegetable shortening, and anything called "cheese product" that is nothing more than coagulated vegetable oil that has been given an artificial color and flavor). Sometimes those unexpected reactions may include inflammation, digestive tract issues (including stomach acid imbalance and bloating), acid reflux, disturbance in the gut microbiome, kidney, liver and gall bladder issues, and bowel irregularity.

Make every effort to eat organic, real food. Avoid manufactured foods, as they likely contain cheap filler ingredients, some of them byproducts of petroleum, which our bodies may be incapable of processing efficiently, possibly resulting in inflammation, discomfort, and allergic reactions, including hives, rashes, digestive ailments, and even seizures. Petro-chemical additives are often simply listed as dyes or "artificial" colors or flavors.

Fruits and vegetables that have been genetically modified may present different risks, especially when the organism was altered to deter natural pests or to make the plant resistant to herbicides. (Euractive)

Processed or Manufactured Foods

Most foods we eat are "processed" in some way. Cooking is a kind of processing. Pickles are processed in brine. Frozen vegetables may be blanched before freezing. Flour is milled. Cucumbers may be sprayed with food-grade wax to increase shelf-life.

When you follow a recipe, you are processing food. When you freeze leftovers, you are processing food. When you dehydrate herbs for your spice shelf, you are processing food.

When a manufacturer does the processing for you, the only real control you have is whether to eat it or not. When food manufacturers add chemicals other than salt to preserve shelf life or enhance flavor, that sort of processing may render the food less nutritious, or harder to digest. The introduction of those chemicals into the body is, at the very least, unnatural. Any food label that has ingredients you do not recognize as something you can buy whole, is worth questioning.

When you are buying something that is premade, ready to eat, you may be eating something that is not only what you think it is. Food manufacturers primarily want profits. This sort of manufactured food might well include cheap ingredients, filler, artificial flavor enhancers, emulsifiers, and/or preservatives to increase shelf life and simply bulk up the product.

Did you know that frozen french fries are often coated with a chemical, often a form of sugar, to help them brown in your oven? Are you aware that when you frequent a chain restaurant that most of that food is likely prepared in a factory and distributed frozen to franchises? If you think you are getting real food from most restaurants, think twice. It may look like real food. It may taste like real food. But you have no idea what's in it.

If a product lists "artificial" flavors or colors, just put it back on the shelf and live well without it. Artificial flavors or colors are often chemically derived as a byproduct of petrochemicals. If you are not sure what that means, it means from crude oil, just like gasoline. In the documentary *Edible City: Grow the Revolution* (Hesse), one of the featured people describes how her daughter suffered petit mal seizures until she removed petrochemicals from her diet. The fact is that we have no control over our food unless we make it ourselves from whole real food ingredients.

If a product lists "natural flavors" as an ingredient and does not specify what those flavors are, you should think it through. The product may or may not be fine, but you should know what you are eating, and under the label "natural flavors," you simply do not know.

The Food and Drug Administration has come under fire in recent years regarding what must be true about a product in order for it to be labeled "natural." In 2016, there was a request for comment from the public. There were lots of expressions of opinion, but there was no consensus on the meaning of the word "natural." Let's just say this: whatever you think "natural" means, it is unlikely that anyone in the FDA, the USDA, the food industry, product marketing, or package design agrees with you. (Center) I tend to think the word is meaningless. (Houck)

I suggest ignoring terms like "natural" and "healthy" altogether and reading the labels and thinking for yourself. If a food product comes with a label, you should read it before you eat it.

Movement

Exercise for many is a dirty word. The entire health-club industry is built on people NOT using their membership. Miracle home exercise gadgets clutter closets and thrift store shelves. How many treadmills, exercycles, and elliptical machines are buried under piles of laundry?

Anyone who has ever used fancy exercise equipment to the point of exhaustion only to learn that they have successfully burned fewer calories than are accounted for in a piece of toast knows the futility of exercising to lose weight and the insanity of counting calories.

Exercise is still important, but let's not call it exercise; let's call it "movement" or "activity." We do not move to burn calories. We move to get from one place to another, to experience new things, to accomplish goals, to get good at moving because moving is fun. Or, at least, it should be and will be.

Movement is important because our physical bodies come with a use-it-or-lose-it quality. The less we move, the harder it becomes to move. It stands to reason, then, that the more we move, the easier it becomes to do so. Movement is part of the harmony of the mind-body connection.

I used to proudly proclaim that I would not run for any reason, not even if someone were chasing me with a knife. I thought running was a sign of allowing life to rile or harry me and I was bound and determined to be a chill guy.

Less than a year into my journey of intermittent fasting and low-carb life, I totaled my car and found myself needing to take two busses to get to my office.

One day, as my first bus had run a bit late, I thought I would miss my connection. Instead, as we arrived, I saw the connecting bus in the next block. Without thinking, I ran and caught the bus. Believe it or not, it was several minutes into that second ride when I realized that I had actually run.

I had been gradually increasing my activity. I had started parking in the far corner of the lot. I started taking the stairs instead of the elevator. I would take a few moments between client visits and stretch or take short walks around the block. And, on that day, my motivation was to get on that bus. I had not thought about it at all. I just ran for it the way I would have when I was a kid. It was only a block. It is not like I ran a mile.

No, I am not training for the next 5K race. I still do not think running is fun. But that is the point. I can run if necessary. So, beyond increasing my activity thinking of it as exercise, it is far better to find movement I genuinely enjoy, even if I get a little winded or have to take it easy at first.

I move to have fun. If I am not good at what I want to do, I move to get better at it and have more fun. Fun, accomplishment, and achievement make up a big part of the mind-body relationship.

Movement increases health, works muscles, harmonizes organs, facilitates the processing of nutrients, increases agility, increases energy, counteracts depression, encourages insulin sensitivity, and even stimulates the brain.

We just need to find out which form of movement we value as fun. That is really the key. Many people think of working out as drudgery, almost a punishment for being fat or out of shape. Instead of seemingly pointless exercise, we would be far better off choosing an activity at which we would like to be good and we think we would enjoy doing. You do not have to be good at it already.

If you find time to watch your favorite show, you have time to do something. Go bowling, take a walk, dance under a sprinkler in the summer heat, make a garden, paint your bedroom, build a shed, help your neighbor with a project, collect scrap metal for extra cash, cut your own grass, or wash your car by hand! If you enjoy lifting weights, then do it. Stop making excuses about why you cannot or do not have time. And if your skill level makes you feel hopeless, determine to get better at whatever it is. If you want to run a marathon, you may have to start by walking around the block. Just move.

You can certainly engage in movement and activity while fasting. If you like working out at a gym, go and do it. Schedule it. Hire a private trainer if you need someone to spot you. All movement, whether you like doing cardio, resistance training, or walking along the beach at sunset, will augment and the benefits of fasting and a LCHF diet. If you have to stay home, then set aside a particular time of day to get active, perhaps with a YouTube trainer.

It is important to remember why we are moving. One of the best times for movement is the morning because if you are experiencing the Dawn Phenomenon, your body is anticipating the need for being awake and moving, so wake up and move.

Remember that it is not about burning calories, but rather taking advantage of the natural functions of the body to eventually establish that new normal. Just remember to stay hydrated, and if you get light-headed, take a break, breathe, and do not overdo it.

The Next Step

You want to continue to increase your natural fast until your average is sixteen to eighteen hours. Stay at this level until your average natural fast reaches at least sixteen hours. If you have difficulty with this process, discuss it with your hypnotist.

Also, you want to consider the carbohydrates that remain in your diet. Until now we have officially cut them by upwards of seventy-five percent. But have you? Are there any more carbohydrates you are now willing to consider cutting? Cut them!

Chapter 8
Stage Five

Food Preferences

Food preferences can be changed. It is not the food but what you think about the food that determines your preferences. If you are an adventurous eater, willing to try almost anything once, then you have a fairly flexible palate. If your palate is limited, nearly anything that does not at least resemble your imagined choices might make you hesitate, and that hesitation comes from the internal monolog that says, "What if I do not like it?" Or worse, "I probably will not like it." Such thoughts are self-fulfilling predictions.

We live life-making predictions like the ones above. Making predictions is actually one of the main purposes for memory. We remember our impressions of people, places, events, circumstances, and conditions and use that information to predict what will happen when the situation is even remotely similar.

The memory/prediction function often works pretty well, but sometimes reality comes with a bit of a shock. In the 1980s, while walking around Chinatown in New York City, I saw a bakery window

79

filled with small, elaborately decorated cakes, about the size of two cupcakes. They looked so good! I imagined the delicious butter-cream frosting and the light, fluffy cake underneath. Imagine my shock and disappointment when I discovered that the frosting was simply colored shortening: no butter, no sugar, no flavor...yuck! For a long time, I had an instinctive distrust of pretty cakes from Asian bakeries.

I have always had an adventurous palate. When I lived in Japan, that palate was seriously challenged when, as a special treat, I was presented with a plate of food that appeared to be moving. It was simply a garnish of shaved, dried fish that moved in the heat of the dish, but it really gave me pause. What I tasted was amazing and actually started a quest to find the best takoyaki in Japan. Everywhere I went, I would get the dish and rate it. Takoyaki is Japanese street food, a kind of pancake ball with a piece of octopus in the middle, garnished with a special sauce and dried seaweed. Yum! If you are interested, the best takoyaki in Japan, in my opinion, was in my hometown of Chiyoda-cho, in Hiroshima prefecture and the second best was in Naha, Okinawa.

On another occasion, a Japanese friend bought me another special street-food treat that set the limits of my adventurous palate. He bought me a palm-sized cooked snail in the shell. I could not get it passed my lips and the aroma completely removed my appetite. My friend, however, slurped it down with great relish.

Here is what I want you to see, and it is important that you see it. No nutritious food is inherently nasty. Andrew Zimmerman from the Travel Channel show *Bizarre Foods* more than adequately demonstrates that point. It is only our impression of the nature of that food that tells us that something is good to eat or not. I was not raised eating snails, but I was raised eating squid. I found the jump to octopus fairly easy while the snail impossible. Perhaps, with increased exposure, I could come to like snails.

Children who dislike vegetables most likely have been taught to dislike vegetables. Dad says he does not like broccoli, or some other kid says, "Yuck!" when peas are on the plate. We may follow their lead, and our choice more reflects our affection for the person than the actual dislike of the food.

Admittedly, there are some things that just do not sit well the first time we try them, even as children, but an adventurous palate can be acquired. My mother insists that I loved green peas as a baby, but as an adult, I dislike them cooked. I love them raw, fresh from the garden, but I avoid the cooked, mushy pustules. (By my phrasing, you can easily note the mental association I have made with that food that many people around the world simply adore.)

I always try peas, and I try to try them with an open mind when they are served in a new way. Sometimes they are innocuous or hardly noticeable. Other times I will actually pick them out of food. Sometimes the dish is so good, I will ask for the recipe. My distaste for plain mushy peas, however, remains. I cannot really blame the vegetable, but rather the methods of preparing it.

Children can also be quite clever. Of course, there are things everyone, a kid included, likes better than others. Some figure out at an incredibly young age that if they refuse to eat long enough, eventually they will get something else that they prefer. They actually cope well with temporary hunger in order to get what they want.

As a hypnotist, I have had several parents bring children who refused to eat anything other than their favorites. One little boy would only eat McDonald's chicken nuggets and fries. It had to be McDonald's, not Burger King, and definitely not frozen nuggets or fries from the grocery store. He knew if he refused to eat long enough, his parents would break down and go and get him McNuggets.

The cure for this problem is not in hypnosis. The parents hoped I could create a desire in their child by snapping my fingers. It does not work that way. Hypnosis can help a *willing* person develop a more adventurous palate, but a person unwilling to change is an unlikely candidate. The actual cure is simple enough. It is not making them sit at the table until they finish their mushy peas. It is not in taking away their electronic games or assigning them a time out.

If they refuse to eat what you are having for dinner, they go hungry. We do not have to bribe children to eat. Hunger is truly the best sauce. A stubborn child will eat long before it gets dangerous. The real trick is keeping Grandma from sneaking the kid McNuggets.

Think of a mom or dad trying to feed a baby in a highchair. At a certain point, the baby begins to turn away from the spoon. It might be that they do not like it, but, really, they have not yet developed much of a palate. Perhaps, just perhaps, the baby no longer feels hunger, but parents somehow believe that the baby needs to eat more. Spoon after spoon gets shoved into that child's mouth, half of it getting spit out again. For heaven's sakes, stop that behavior. A hungry child will eat! And force-feeding a child who does not feel hungry only plants seeds of eating problems, like not stopping when they are full.

In the documentary *The Magic Pill* (Tate), a little girl with a very picky palate completely changed. The parents speak very frankly about their experience, their fears, even anxiety and emotional pain of not giving in to their daughter's childish stubborn palate. If you are struggling with a picky child, I recommend that documentary.

Of course, consult your pediatrician but ultimately the answer may in your education and a concerted effort on the part of the whole family.

Natural, Healthy, or Organic

Any manufactured food that is labeled "natural" or "healthy" is immediately suspect; the food manufacturer's labels mean extraordinarily little. They are simply a marketing ploy to get you to feel better about a product.

If a product is labeled "USDA Organic," no pesticides were used to grow the ingredients and the seeds were non-GMO. If meat or eggs are labeled organic, it means that those animals were fed food that was certified organic. It is probably still grain, but at least it is organic grain. In terms of chicken or eggs, free-range means little, while pasture-raised means a lot. Free range for chickens and eggs basically means the animals were not kept in cages. It does not mean they were out on pasture, eating bugs and grass, but were likely kept in a vast warehouse on the ground eating feed.

Much of the fresh produce in the United States cannot be labeled "organic" because of pesticides and genetically modified seeds. Most genetically modified veggies were modified to increase shelf life, improve sturdiness for shipping, or be resistant to herbicides, which allows the farmer to chemically kill weeds without damaging the crop. This herbicide, often glyphosate, to which certain GMO plants are resistant, appears in the food we eat. The dangers of glyphosate, a probable carcinogen, are even made worse by the inert ingredients that deliver it. (Charles) (Gammon)

In general, except for corn, vegetables that can be peeled have reduced added pesticide exposure. The highest exposure to pesticides comes from sprayed pesticides on vegetables that we do not peel, like leafy greens.

Corn is obviously shucked, but there is a difference because the pesticide "bacillus thuringiensis," a naturally occurring fungus in soil, has been spliced into the genome of the corn. When bugs eat it, they die. Originated by Monsanto, now Bayer, a three-month Monsanto-sponsored study in rats demonstrated that it's "safe" for human consumption. However, when the same study was replicated in France over a six-month period, the rats developed severe tumors. (Euractive)

Currently, about 92% of the corn in the United States is "Bt-Corn." This means the corn itself and all the products derived from corn (corn chips, cereals, starch, corn-syrup, other food additives) are made from pesticide-laced corn. Bon appetit!

Along those lines, 94% of soybeans are genetically modified, and therefore, the products from soy are similarly changed.

Here is a question I would like to propose. Given the presence of glyphosates in our vegetables. Given the fact that we know that when we consume meat from livestock that has been fed antibiotics, we contribute to the development and susceptibility to antibiotic-resistant strains of bacterial infection. Could the burgeoning numbers of people who suffer from celiac disease (a form of gluten intolerance), Crohn's disease, irritable bowel syndrome, leaky gut syndrome, ulcerative colitis, or any other digestive tract issues, be attributed to our adulterated food supply?

The problem with labels is that we pay for them. Things labeled "natural" or "healthy" sell better because they are not as expensive as organic products, and people think they are still better than regular products, which may or may not be true.

What we need to do is to make the best buying decisions based on our budgets and an educated read of the ingredient and nutrition labels.

Hands down, grass fed, grass-finished meat that come from animals that were humanely slaughtered are the best. Similarly, full-fat dairy products (milk, cheese, yogurt, cream) that come from grass fed, grass-finished cows, sheep, or goats are of better quality for not being tainted with antibiotics or unnatural grain food. (Cows do not eat corn naturally. They eat grass.) However, these products can be quite expensive.

Our job is to get the best quality real food for the money that we have to spend. Some of us choose to eat less of something in order to afford a higher quality product. Some give up on certain products entirely. And for the rest, we buy the best we can afford at the time. And some of us actually choose to grow much of our own produce.

Ingredient Labels

We have already considered some ingredients that might make someone decide not to buy a product. Hidden sugar under its various names and chemically extracted oils can be problem ingredients. They have a negative impact on the microbiome in your digestive system, can cause inflammation, and/or inhibit or fail to provide nutritive value.

Chemical flavor enhancers, artificial colors, and artificial flavors make some processed foods more appealing, but at the cost of ingesting petrochemicals. Artificial sweeteners have demonstrated both chemical risks, including nerve damage, and for triggering cephalic insulin response, ultimately negating any value they may have provided.

Eliminating just these three groups would very nearly wipe out all the groceries in the middle of the store and many on the perimeter, especially in the dairy section. You might find yourself looking for land to homestead to grow your own food.

Let's get real and honest here. Do the best you can. You may choose to learn to cook some things from scratch rather than buying premade products. You may choose to spend more on better premade products. You may just have to do the best you can on the budget you have. I do not endorse irrational fanaticism. I simply buy the best I can afford using the information I have. If I am doing the best I can do, that is really the best I can do. It is unlikely that you will be able to eliminate all the ingredients that you would like without spending a lot of money and a lot of time in the kitchen.

As for the key to reading ingredient labels, know that they are listed in decreasing order of predominance. That means that the first ingredient on the list represents the biggest portion of the product and the last ingredient listed represents the tiniest portion.

That says NOTHING about the impact of that ingredient. Of course, if the first ingredient is sugar, rethink the product. But also consider that sugar may be listed under several names making the overall sugar content even higher.

That decision is yours. But, as you proceed in your new lifestyle, you may come to determine that certain ingredients can and should be avoided at any cost. I will not, for example, eat corn that is not certified organic. The truth is, corn is a grain and eating it at all is extremely rare for me; because of how it has been genetically modified, I just do not want that chemistry in my body. I might nibble a few puffs of organic popcorn and may once or twice a season have an ear of organic corn on the cob.

Nutrition Labels

The Hypnofasting Program is mostly concerned with three items on a nutrition label: serving size, carbohydrates, and fiber. We ignore the calories, and, in terms of macronutrients, we ignore the percent of daily value.

Notice the "per serving" caveat. One of the tasks I recommend is to take several of your preferred products and measure out a single serving. Then compare that single serving to what they would normally eat. You may need to use a kitchen scale or a set of measuring spoons and cups. If the serving size indicates one tablespoon, it is a level not a heaping tablespoon.

A digital kitchen scale is a good investment. It does not have to be expensive to work. Whether the serving size is expressed in ounces, grams, or some other measure, understanding what a single serving means is critical. Also, many recipes you might try along your Hypnofasting Program journey might be expressed in grams. Placing an empty bowl on the scale, pressing the "tare" button, zeros out the weight so you can accurately measure your ingredients.

Take a moment to get from your pantry a product with a nutrition label. It does not matter what it is. In the U.S., the label is standardized.

Notice the serving size near the top expressed in size or grams or both. Measure it out to see what it looks like. You will quickly notice that your regular consumption patterns far exceed the single portion size.

Unless you are a vegetarian or vegan and need to calculate your macronutrient percentages, you can happily skip over the calorie content.

We can skip total, saturated, and trans-fat because we have already read the ingredient label. We have learned that saturated fat is not as scary as we have been taught. And we are already avoiding poly-unsaturated fats. If you see trans-fat listed, read the ingredients label again. You will find the words "hydrogenated" or "partially hydrogenated" listed along with some really bad oil.

Skip cholesterol and the sodium. We just do not need that information. If you are concerned about cholesterol because of the risk to cardiovascular health, triglycerides have been demonstrated to be more indicative of risk. You may want to discuss your triglycerides with your physician. If you are concerned about sodium because of the possible effects on your blood pressure, know that not only has salt been unfairly framed as the culprit, and there are also natural ways of lowering your blood pressure. (Berry, Why Salt)

Consider the total carbohydrate listing. It is expressed in grams. (If you were a strict ketogenic diet person, you would keep carbohydrates to less than 10% of your diet.) That may be a choice for you later, but in The Hypnofasting Program, we refrain from setting such objectives, except perhaps on an individual basis.

Under the total carbohydrates listing, you should see a number for dietary fiber, another for sugars (notice the plural) and another for added sugars.

Subtract the dietary fiber from the total carbohydrate, and you arrive at the net carbohydrate number. This is the information we want to think about because it indicates that we will be triggering the production of insulin. The lower the number of net carbs, the better. If you end up counting carbohydrates, the net number is what you use.

But, make no mistake, carbs are not eliminated by fiber. Those carbohydrates still exist, but the fiber makes for a better balance and a more controlled insulin reaction.

Now notice something else. Notice how much of the total sugars are actually "added sugars." This means that they simply spooned in the sugar, or corn syrup or dextrose or whatever sugar product was cheapest and fit the flavor profile.

Just understanding nutrition labels will help you make better buying decisions. We are looking for foods that are lower in carbohydrates and higher in fiber per serving. Remember if you consume more than one serving, these numbers multiply. Fiber is a prebiotic, meaning that our microbiome likes fiber. Fiber also counters some of the carbohydrate content.

You may already be taking a probiotic supplement. Your gut microbiome is important and should be nurtured. Monitoring the regularity of your bowel movements is important to understand your microbiome. A good, multi-strain probiotic supplement may be in order.

Purging and Shopping

You can, of course, completely purge your cabinets and fridge of everything undesirable, but you will find yourself with empty cabinets and spending a lot of money fast because of a change that you may ultimately find unsustainable.

Instead of a grand purge, choose one or two products from your pantry. Read the ingredient and nutrition labels. Based on what you have learned, do you think you will purchase those products again when your supply runs out? Be sane about your pantry.

There will be some things that you simply decide to throw away and live without. We all do it, but it is more likely that in the interim, while you are depleting your supplies of that product, that you will look for, or create better, more nutritious replacements.

Pick a product—say, a condiment, like ketchup, mayonnaise, or relish. Get it and read both the ingredient list and the nutritional label. Is there anything on the ingredient label you do not want to eat? How carbohydrate-laden is this product? How much do you normally use, and how does that compare to the suggested serving size?

A Moving Experience

We know that movement is important, and in the last stage, I asked you to think about something you could do to move more and have fun. Did you pick something? What steps have you taken to implement the movement?

It does not have to be difficult. It could be as simple as walking the dog instead of letting her mess up the backyard. Perhaps parking at spaces more distant to the front door of the store. Taking the stairs instead of the elevator. Or dancing with the broom as you sweep the floor.

Whatever you are doing, you need to be consistent in doing it long enough that your body comes to believe that this new movement is becoming normal.

If you have not yet found an activity that suits you, do not wait. Do something! You can always change your mind later and pick something new. In fact, you probably will, but that is OK, too. I recently met a woman who described signing up for snowboarding lessons. She thought she might like the activity because she liked to ski. In one lesson she realized that she did not enjoy the activity as much as she thought she would.

Activities that are prosocial are often more rewarding than those you do alone. It may not be enough to join a spin class and go. Instead, take the time to make new acquaintances that might just develop into positive friendships. If the activities you choose are prosocial, you will more likely look forward to going, less likely to talk yourself out of going, and you will enjoy the activity more.

If you prefer to be alone, that is OK, too. Just be vigilant about being active long enough to see your own improvement. The alone factor is one of the biggest reasons people keep buying home exercise equipment but then never use it.

Your First OMAD

OMAD stands for One Meal a Day. Now that your natural fast is averaging sixteen to eighteen hours, we are ready to begin our intermittent fasting regimen.

What's that? You thought you were fasting? Nope, not yet. Now the fun begins. For hypnofasters, the days that have a six-to-eight-hour eating window are actually our *feasting* days, not fasting days. Of course, there will occasionally be days where you cut your natural fast short for some hopefully legitimate reason, but we do not intend that to be a habit. I know a woman who never eats a morning meal except on Saturday when she and her husband do a full breakfast together. (Forget the pancakes and the toast.) She makes a keto bread for dipping into her egg yolks and fries their eggs in the fat from the bacon. They enjoy a side of mushrooms and spinach sauteed in butter and drizzled with a creamy garlic sauce she makes from scratch. For her, unless she eats early on Friday evening, her natural fast is shortened most Saturdays.

From this point forward, what we will call our intermittent fasting days will all be 24 hours or longer. Do not let that scare you. It is easier than you imagine, and those days will now become intermittent or irregular. It is difficult to eat enough in a single meal to sustain your metabolism. Take this as a warning because many hypnofasters find OMAD to be fairly comfortable, and the danger of making it a standard practice is real, and it is too soon in our process to do anything that establishes a repeated pattern.

Social media is full of stories of people who have plateaued on LCHF or ketogenic diets, and most often, we find they have an extremely limited understanding of the role of intermittent fasting and what it really means.

If a fast of twenty-four-plus hours sounds extreme to you, remember that we are resetting what your brain-body considers normal. In order to do that, we must keep from establishing a consistent eating pattern while maintaining a minimum standard of natural fasting so that our brain-body mechanism does establish a new normal.

After a twenty-four-hour fast, most people will have used up the glycogen stored in their liver and may have already begun converting fat to energy. If you have not lost much weight yet, OMAD will certainly help.

OMAD sounds tough. It really is not as hard as it sounds, but let's talk about some of the things that you can do to complete your first OMAD.

You are almost there anyway. You have probably worked your way up to eighteen or twenty hours. It is just a few more hours.

Plan your fast. Pick the day and time to begin and end your OMAD. Choose days that you expect to be busy. Perhaps finish eating a little early on the day you begin your fast. Tell yourself that you can eat any time after that same time the next day. Be careful not to phrase your plan as "I cannot eat until." That is counterproductive, and you are much less likely to be successful. Instead, use "I'll eat any time after…"

Plan your next meal. Know what and how much you will eat when you break your fast. Stick to proteins and fats for that first meal. It is better to avoid carbohydrates when breaking a fast because of the rapid spike in blood sugar.

Keep busy. The more your mind is occupied, the less you will think about food. It is a great time to start cleaning the basement, garage, or attic.

Stay hydrated. Drink water. You can make water more interesting by adding a little salt, apple cider vinegar, or a squeeze of lemon or lime. Of course, black coffee, unsweetened tea, and herbal teas are always good choices. If you think you are not going to make it, a cup of good bone broth will help get you through, particularly during your first few OMADs.

Diabetics: monitor your blood sugar. Keep in mind that if you are taking certain diabetes medications, fasting for twenty-four hours may result in low blood sugar levels. Know the symptoms and have food or juice handy just in case.

If you have not already formed a plan to reduce your diabetes medications, now is a good time to consult your physician. I cannot stress this enough.

When you break your fast, eat a well-portioned meal. Remember to eat both intentionally and mindfully. Eat until you are full, then stop. Many people discover they cannot finish their plate. Depending on the time of your first meal, feel free to eat another meal several hours later.

The Carbs That Remain

The question now is very simply, are they worth it? Remembering that carbohydrates, especially processed carbohydrates, cause the biggest spike to blood glucose levels, triggering insulin and perhaps slowing or even halting gluconeogenesis, ask yourself if that cracker, noodle, or even breading on a piece of chicken is worth the consequences before you reach your goal.

Carbohydrates offer little to no nutritive value and carry no nutrients that you cannot get from otherwise nutrient dense foods. What is their purpose now?

You are the only one who can make that decision, but by now, your cravings for carbohydrates are conceivably under control. Now carbohydrates are more in perspective than they once were. Though you have always been the one to decide what you eat and do not eat in this program, you are now in a better position to make an educated decision about those foods and size of the role they play in your diet.

Well-Intentioned Opposition

Let's face it. In our society, not eating is not normal. Often when we meet friends, our activities involve eating. Unless we live alone, we probably share, prepare, and eat food regularly with others. When we are at work, we congregate around coffee stations and vending machines or break rooms.

Eating together is something humans have been doing for thousands of years, and on occasion, you will be breaking that tradition. People may be uncomfortable if you are not eating with them. If you are a parent, you may have always tried to eat with the kids. Your family will notice that you are not eating. Often, saying "I'm just not hungry" is reason enough. It is good to teach the kids that it is OK to not eat when you are not hungry.

It is not a lie. If we see hunger as a condition and not merely a desire to eat, you are not hungry. You have enough stored energy on your body to get you through. You may be feeling hunger. You may be tempted to taste the food or have just a little, but you know it would interrupt the benefits of your program, so just say, "I am not hungry." And if they insist, resist. On more than one occasion, I have merely shrugged my shoulders and said, "I am allowed to not eat if I don't want to eat."

They will pry, ask all sorts of questions, express concern for your health, suggest you are starving yourself, and, as they see your progress, they will wonder and perhaps ask if you are sick, even suggesting you see a doctor, especially if they have not seen you for a while and you have visibly lost weight.

If you are out with friends and you had not planned on eating at that time, you do not have to. They will ask why you are not eating. Again, the answer is "I am not hungry."

They will say they feel uncomfortable if you are not eating. It is not your duty to make someone feel more comfortable about eating in front of you. Assure them of your companionship and your own comfort. "Oh, please enjoy your meal. I'm enjoying your company. I am not hungry. If I eat now, I will not appreciate it and I will feel uncomfortable." The last bit of the sentence is important because it places them in the position of making you uncomfortable if they force you to eat. That usually ends the cajoling.

Of course, if you are sitting at the table staring longingly at their platter of nachos, your credibility will be severely compromised. If it happens, smile, and say, "That looks really good. I wish I could eat, but honestly…" (hand to your stomach), "I couldn't take a bite." You do not have to explain why you cannot take a bite.

I have had friends actually order food for me, and I have taken it home. "I wish I could eat this now, but I just can't. Thank you for understanding. I'll save this for later." I never promise to eat it, especially if it is loaded with carbohydrates.

I had friends give me trays of cookies at holiday time and ask if I liked them. My answer? "They were delicious." Perhaps I gave them to someone else who said they were delicious, or I simply tossed them out and knew that they would be delicious.

It just takes a while for them to get used to the fact that you are with them for their company, not the food. This is a great time to add dimension to your relationship. Do something fun, perhaps something that involves an activity or movement.

There were a few friends with whom I eventually shared my journey and got some unexpected results.

Some of my friends who are diabetic thought I was criticizing them for what they were eating. One of them seems to think she needs to justify her food choices by telling me how her blood glucose is under control. Another proclaims how much weight he has lost doing it his way. I just smile and take his word for it. I have to take his word for it as there is no other evidence of any weight loss.

It is no secret that a LCHF diet and intermittent fasting are still a bit uncommon and seen as fads. After all, based on the USDA and FDA recommendations, we should be grazing on refined carbohydrates all day long. However, we have taken the time to look at the research, understand the societal pressures, and, finally, take control of our own experiences in life.

What most do not understand is that we are not dieting. We are changing our lives. We are establishing a new normal way of living. In gently but firmly asserting your right to not eat, you are taking control of another aspect of your mind-body. You are demonstrating self-respect, self-esteem, and autonomy.

Joseph A. Onesta

Chapter 9
Stage Six

Genetic Destiny?

When DNA was first defined, there was great hope that science would decode human DNA and thus be able to predict, prevent, and perhaps even cure many illnesses.

What we learned from the actual decoding of the human genome is that humans have far fewer genes than were suspected, and the system was far more complex and interrelated than we hoped. There did not seem to be enough genes to manage the complexity of a human being. Science had to reconsider how it thought about genes.

This interrelatedness was really good news because the prospect of having specific genes responsible for every aspect of our being meant that freedom of choice might not really exist and there might not be much room for self-determination. The good news is that we are not locked into a genetic destiny.

Society generally labels obese people as lazy or lacking in willpower. I, like many obese people, dieted on and off all my life. I struggled all my life. While society blamed me, I knew I was trying my best and I was objectively exercising more willpower than most skinny people. Genetics is one of the excuses some people use to deflect that judgment.

It may be convenient to blame obesity or diabetes on inherited qualities, but it is not as simple as that. While we can look at family groups who share similar body types, and it seems that obesity might run in the family, it is far more likely that obesity has multiple contributing factors beyond any genetic predisposition. Customs, culture, economic status, social pressure, and food culture are much more potent.

Do you always have to clean your plate? Were you bribed with sweets as a child? Does your ethnic background emphasize some foods over others? Did you grow up eating frozen prepared foods, fast food, or in family-style restaurants? Did you eat well-rounded meals together or did everyone grab something quick on the run? Were your parents good cooks? Was your home typically filled with junk food, snacks, and treats?

What about the activity environment in which you grew up? Did your family go on hikes, take bike rides, or encourage sports? Or did your family activities revolve around going to the movies, eating popcorn, and drinking soda pop? Sometimes even simple things make a difference. What kind of chores were your responsibility as a youngster? Did you cut the grass with a push mower or a riding mower, or did your family pay someone else to do it? When I was a teenager, I cut the grass for several neighbors, and in the winter, a heavy snowfall was an opportunity to brandish a shovel and go around the neighborhood earning pocket money for clearing sidewalks and driveways.

Food and movement environments are far more indicative of obesity than genetics. While genes play a part in our predispositions, the science of epigenetics demonstrates that genes interact with their environment. Even if you think you are genetically predisposed to put on the pounds or are susceptible to insulin resistance, you can do something about it by controlling your environment. It seems that genes have a kind of dial that changes what they do, almost an on/off switch. (Lipton)

So, even if you are somehow predisposed to insulin resistance or obesity, you can counter that predisposition by changing the food and activity environment in which you live. But, we also have to understand that we live in a cultivated, social food environment that is essentially profit motivated, and more importantly, very unhealthy, especially when that social environment inaccurately promotes itself as being healthy.

We cannot entirely blame the epidemic of obesity and type 2 diabetes on genetics, and it is essentially unfair to blame an individual in our social food environment for those conditions. The irony, of course, is that while we might campaign to change attitudes, conventions, or even regulated food policies, the real responsibility for learning and taking control of wellness sits firmly in the lap of individuals like you and me. And as we individually join that barbarian horde at the gate of profit-driven agriculture, husbandry, processed food and pharmacological industries, we engender and cultivate the change that inevitably will take place.

Metabolism

Have you ever driven a car that when you took your foot off the break, moved forward, even without your taping the gas? If so, the "idle" of your car was high. That means that your car burned a higher amount of fuel even when it was standing still. Think of your metabolism as your body's idle.

You still burn energy when you sit quietly doing nothing. You even burn energy when you are asleep. If you believe you have a slow metabolism, you may be right, especially if you have yo-yo dieted, followed reduced-calorie diets, or followed any restrictive diet for a significant period of time.

Your success depends on establishing a new normal, for your mind, brain and body. This requires an adjustment to your metabolism. In effect, we want to turn up your idle. To do so, you need to eat well, that is, eat wholesome, nutrient-dense, real food. It also means keeping your movement and activity levels high enough to essentially keep your engine in good working order. And it means retraining your mind to perceive and expect a higher level of wellness.

Avoid supplements that promise an increased metabolism. Shun energy drinks and over-the-counter diet pills or supplements. They are a waste of your money and are a concoction of chemicals can negatively affect your system. If your doctor has prescribed a diet pill, take time to actually read what the medication is, what it does, and what the side effects might be. Also learn how to stop using it. A diet pill is not an ideal part of your new normal.

The best way to actually change your metabolism is both to eat good nutrient dense food and tune up your body through activity. Your body knows what it needs in order to do what you do. If you consume extra, your body knows how to store away reserves. By gradually changing your diet and activity levels, your body will adjust your metabolism automatically.

Metabolic disease is not merely a function of the habits of the individual but is a predictable outcome of some of the societal trends that have taken place within the last sixty years. Our cultural diet has moved from fresh meat and vegetables prepared at home for family meals to highly processed food products, industrialized food production that depends on broad-scale mono-culture farming and husbandry, which relies heavily on government-subsidies to produce carbohydrates, mostly from grains.

Americans extract an astonishing number of byproducts from GMO corn and soy. Most of it is used as animal feed and cheap filler ingredients. Industrialized meat is produced by feeding grain to a large number of animals because there could never be enough grazing for that many animals—yet it is perfectly *unnatural* for a cow to eat corn. Chickens have been bred to grow so fast on their grain diet that many actually perish under their own weight. Because of the artificial, close, movement-limiting environment in which these animals are raised, they need antibiotics just to remain healthy long enough to make it to slaughter. (Pearce)

While extremely profitable for the food industries, it is not ideal for health and wellness. The excuse the food industry asserts to justify industrial methods is that organic agriculture and husbandry are inefficient to the point that we would not be able to provide food for our population.

Stop right there. How is that true when upwards of 40% of the food produced in the United States does not make it to market? Forty percent of the food produced in this country goes to landfill (USDA), and yet, upwards of one in five children in this country go to bed hungry or subsist on cheap, subsidized, sugar-filled junk "food." (Gregory) Because of that pseudo food, many more children go to bed undernourished.

Indeed, organic farming is sustainable. It just is not as profitable as industrialized agricultural practices. Industrialized agriculture is designed to win the price wars against sustainable organic farming, leaving the organic farmer to market produce for high prices only in elite markets. (Hasse)

The epidemic proportions of obesity and diabetes in our country has been cultivated, perhaps unintentionally, but cultivated all the same. Still endorsed by the USDA in its design of the food recommendations historically through the food pyramid (which has been replaced by "My Plate," which recommends that more than 50% of diet comes from insulin-stimulating, liver-taxing carbohydrates). (Choose)

If you follow those guidelines, your chance of becoming obese and/or developing type 2 diabetes, both of which have skyrocketed in the last sixty years, seems significantly higher. That is the societal environment in which your metabolism has been cultivated. While I have no doubt that the food industry lobby played a major backroom part in establishing the standards, I will not suggest that the motive was malicious. I would, however, suggest that in the advent of better food science, profit was and remains more of a concern than feeding hungry people. Otherwise, all that food that is tossed into the landfill would find its way to those hungry children.

Those of us who have fallen into the obesity and or diabetes vortex, and indeed, all of us, need to learn to think for ourselves, understand our bodies, and do what we need to do to achieve wellness and sustain our health as much as we can. Let's thank the government and industry for the offer to help, but let's move forward a bit more consciously, and when it comes to industrial food, a bit more skeptically.

There are two classically understood aspects to metabolism: diet and exercise, what we now call movement or activity. There is a third aspect, which is commonly neglected: mindset.

In The Hypnofasting Program, when I say "diet," I am not talking about calories, but nutrition. When I say "movement," I am not talking about working out at the gym, but general, overall levels of movement or activity. When I say "mindset," I am really talking about attitudes and mindfully monitoring our internal monologue.

The brain-body tends to stabilize based on average long-standing patterns. That is what we had been doing up until beginning The Hypnofasting Program created our old normal. Since beginning this program, we have upset those patterns, making it difficult for the brain-body to settle in. Our metabolism changes when our average nutritive intake and our average activity levels establish a new long-term pattern. It does not take much imagination to understand that if we go back to doing what we had been doing before The Hypnofasting Program, we will just go back to our old normal.

We have already talked about how a reduced calorie diet damages our metabolism. Reduced calories for an extended period of time causes our brain-body to adjust its efficiency based on average caloric intake. It senses lean times and behaves accordingly by tightening its energy expense belt, the way we might tighten our purse strings during a temporary financial crisis.

By shifting our macronutrient mix, we are giving the brain-body sufficiently different information to upset the balance. By eating more nutrient-dense food, our system is no longer sorting through a lot of empty calories to find what it needs. By moving more, we cause our brain-body to hormonally adjust and more freely use the fuel we have stored and later, consume. In adjusting our perceptions and expectations, we create an environment for wellness allowing natural epigenetic responses to take place.

We will examine these aspects of metabolism in greater detail in the next stage.

Three Staggered OMADs

In this stage, while maintaining a regular daily fasting regimen of sixteen to eighteen hours and a regular eating window of six to eight hours, conduct three OMAD fasts in succession. We will eat just one meal a day for three days in a row but stagger the times we eat.

On the first day, eat breakfast, even if it means your previous natural fast was cut short. After you finish your breakfast, eat nothing again until *lunch* the next day. Yes, it is a bit longer than an OMAD, but there is rhyme to my reasoning. Let's call it OMAD *plus*. After you finish your lunch, eat nothing again until dinner the following day. That is your second OMAD *plus*. After you finish dinner, eat nothing again until dinner the next day. This is your third OMAD. After you finish your dinner, do not eat again until after your natural fast of sixteen to eighteen hours has passed. Then eat as is your custom on non-fasting, natural fast days.

As long as you remain at this current stage, complete this pattern of OMADs every week just change your starting day to mix things up. Here are some helpful fasting reminders:

- Stay hydrated and get enough salt.
- Avoid carbohydrates in the meals that break your fast.
- Plan the meal that will break your fast.
- Stay busy and keep your mind occupied.
- Monitor your internal monologue.
- Acknowledge and observe feelings of hunger and how they pass.
- Drink as much as you want. (Berry, What you)
- If you really think you cannot make it, have a cup of good quality bone broth, preferably at the twenty-four-hour mark, then eat nothing until the meal you have scheduled. You can make it; it is just a few hours longer.

Carbs You "Couldn't" Give Up

Until now, all the choices have been yours. Technically, they still are, but will you allow me to push you just a bit? Let me tell you why.

In my own journey, I came to realize that some of the limitations I set early in the process no longer seemed critical. Things began to change. I discovered that some of the foods, carbohydrates mostly, that I had once thought were impossible to live without, no longer mattered. I could sit at a picnic table, watching people gnaw their way through ear after ear of corn, without much difficulty. I could sing "Happy Birthday" without anticipating cake. After trying many keto bread recipes, some of them were quite good, but I just was not eating them.

About the time that I was reaching this point in my journey, a client came to see me about abating a driving phobia. He had a lot of anxiety anytime he drove a car. In our hypnosis session, I asked his unconscious mind to take him to a time in his life when he conquered a fear. The ability to conquer a fear is a resource we hypnotists help clients apply to other situations and circumstances. I will summarize his story here.

During the summer he turned thirteen, he spent several weeks with relatives. On hot afternoons, he and his cousins would go to a swimming hole in a very slow-moving river nearby. In the middle of the river, where the water was deepest, there was an old stone pylon that had once supported a bridge that had been dismantled when a newer bridge was erected downstream. The top of the pylon hovered some twenty feet above the surface of the water. His cousins would scale the pylon and jump into the water, and they dared him to do it. When they saw he was afraid, they teased him and cajoled him into trying.

"You do not know how high twenty feet is until you are looking down at dark water. Climbing up the metal rungs, I just looked straight at the stone, I couldn't look down. But when I got up there and saw how high we were, I could not move. I was frozen. I started to shake. I could not even think of climbing back down.

So my cousin Benny shoved me off. I cursed him all the way down. I was a little surprised at how hard the water felt from that height, and how deep I went before coming back to the surface, but it was kind of fun. After that, I did it on my own. Jumped and jumped. It was a great vacation."

If you are wondering what this story has to do with cutting carbohydrates, I will explain. I never dreamed that I could ever not crave, much less rarely if ever, eat certain foods. I loved corn on the cob. Cake was a real weakness for me. Bread and pasta were part of my daily life. I never thought I could live happily without them. But I do.

So, I want to challenge you. Push you off the pylon, so to speak.

Are there any carbohydrates or sugary foods you thought, or may still think, you cannot live without? I challenge you to avoid at least one of these items for the next week or so just to see how you do.

You may discover that you do not need them as much as you thought you did. Even more to the point, you might discover that you actually do not want them as much as you thought you did.

Diabetes Medications

Diabetes medications are designed to manage blood glucose levels because persistent high glucose causes neuronal damage and may result in tissue necrosis requiring amputation. Because there is so much glucose in the blood, cells try to avoid consuming it because they do not need it. Because type 2 diabetics and prediabetics are insulin resistant, it takes more insulin to do the job.

There are two forms of prescribed insulin, and those using them have to monitor their blood glucose levels frequently and inject the appropriate kind and amount of insulin to manage their blood glucose levels. They know that injecting too much, or the wrong kind of insulin, can be dangerous.

Some medications called "sulfonylureas" increase the body's own production of insulin. On a low-carb diet combined with intermittent fasting, both direct insulin and sulfonylureas can cause low blood sugar levels with some profoundly serious consequences. If you have been following the program thus far, your medication doses have probably been changed, except perhaps for Metformin.

Metformin, the most common medication for diabetes, especially early cases, inhibits the release of glucose from the liver. If you have not really examined the medications you are taking, how they work, and their possible side effects, you should take the time to do so.

Since Metformin is really inhibiting the release of glucose from the liver, it may now or at some time in the near future impede your weight loss. We want our liver to begin to access fat, convert it into glucose (and later ketones), and release it into the bloodstream to be used as fuel for our bodies.

I am not telling you to stop taking Metformin or any of your medications. That decision must be made in consultation with your doctor. If your doctor agrees to remove Metformin from your regimen, you may not notice any change for three or four days. That is how long Metformin remains in your system. After that period, you may notice an elevation in your blood glucose readings, especially during the Dawn Phenomenon.

The elevation in blood glucose is actually good news in the short term. It means your liver is doing its job. Increase your movement, monitor your blood glucose levels, and keep your doctor informed.

Joseph A. Onesta

Chapter 10
Stage Seven

In the previous stage, we looked at metabolism in a general way. I took the liberty of adding mindset to the traditionally recognized elements of diet and movement and defined the three terms. Let me remind you of those definitions. Diet means nutrition, not calories. Movement is general activity levels, not necessarily working out at a gym. Mindset is made up of the perceptions and expectations of wellness especially as it pertains to our internal monologue.

By considering each aspect of metabolism in a little more detail, we can begin to better understand metabolism and apply that understanding to resetting it...creating our new normal.

Nutrition and Metabolism

Remember that when someone goes on a reduced calorie diet, the body adjusts its energy usage, effectively lowering the metabolism. We can successfully avoid this natural tendency to ration energy in lean times as long as we eat sufficient quantities of nutrient-dense food. I hesitate to use the word calories here because it's not merely about calories—it's about nutrients. Some do consume fewer calories, but others actually increase their caloric intake, especially if they have been watching their caloric intake for a long time.

Remember, we are looking for the new normal. That new normal may require a different caloric intake. What is critical is that calorie for calorie, we are consuming nutrient dense foods. Our bodies no longer have to search through untold quantities of nutrient-sparse and often nutrient-empty calories, looking for what it needs.

When our bodies have the proper nutrients, we can eat until we are satisfied. Grehelin (increases appetite) and leptin (decreases appetite) will begin to function and interact properly.

If we eat real, whole food rich in meat, protein, and above-ground vegetables, (with perhaps some very moderate carbohydrates) we will be getting the nutrients we need.

The brain-body will eventually catch up with the shift from the old normal to the new. While there may be some extenuating conditions, the body will adjust and regulate its hormones appropriately—not only ghrelin and leptin, but insulin, too.

Remember that I promised that you will have some wiggle room, but by the time you have it, you will be less inclined to want to wiggle.

When your new normal is really your normal, you will crave carbohydrates less. Imagine being able to pass by a rack of candy bars or walk through the chip and snacks aisle at the grocery store and not even be tempted. Not many people can do that, but it will become natural for you.

Indeed, some clients report no longer being tempted, and those who choose to occasionally indulge find that it is no indulgence at all or one that is even more precious because of its rarity. One client told me of longing after a piece of pizza, and he decided that he could have a slice. (And he could, of course.) "It was my favorite pizza shop, but it was not the same. I kept thinking, what is wrong with this pizza?

Then it dawned on me that the pizza had not changed, but I had. I did not bother finishing it."

Not everyone will shun carbohydrates completely. I live in Pittsburgh, and we have a local tradition called a cookie table. Whenever there are large events, graduation parties, weddings, family reunions, that sort of thing, the home bakers go into action. When you arrive at a Pittsburgh celebration, there is a large table filled with the most delicious looking homemade cookies. Most people get a plate and stack it high with delectable delights and nibble on them until the meal is served. In Pittsburgh, cookies are a big deal, and that cookie table is a deep-seated tradition. Another client, recounting her nephew's graduation party, said, "I stood there and pondered which one I wanted. Mind you, which ONE!"

Let me give you my own example. We have an apple tree in our yard. This year I went out to pick some apples because I wanted to try to make my own apple cider vinegar. Insect damage makes using these apples a real chore. I have to cut out the wormy bits. But I found one truly pristine, magnificently ripe apple. I had not eaten fresh fruit for over a year because of the fructose, and I want my liver to fully recover from the years of carbohydrate abuse it had suffered. I considered that apple. It was fresh, obviously in season, and only one. I stopped everything I was doing, and I ate that apple both intentionally and mindfully. It was delightful, sweet, and juicy. When I finished it, I was fully satisfied. For a moment, I considered looking for another one but I knew no second apple, even if I found another pristine one, would be better than the first. I really enjoyed that apple, and I felt as if I had been given a gift. (I tested my blood glucose out of curiosity an hour later. It was 102, if you are curious.)

Most of us do not know what it means to eat sufficient quantities of nutrient-dense food. Most of what we have consumed over the years has been nutrient-sparse, empty, or artificially "enriched" (with nutrients we might not even be able to absorb). Think about why a food manufacturer would want to "enrich" any product. The nutrient label would otherwise reveal that the product has no nutritive value. You think you are buying food, but it really is just empty calories sprayed with vitamins. Manufacturers will gladly coat even garbage with chemicals and call it *enriched* if doing so convinces you that it is good for you and you buy it.

The nutritional supplement industry enjoys the nutritional scarcity in our processed food. It is almost instinctual to want to run out and get a bunch of vitamin supplements. Do not do that. You are not going to reset your metabolism with a pill. As you experience changes in your body, you really should become aware of your body's need for vitamins and minerals, and you should be willing to learn about the vitamin and mineral content in the food you eat. If you think supplements are in order, please learn before you buy, or at least before you buy again.

There are some nutrients that are commonly lacking in our cultural diet. If you think you need a supplement, you should know why you need it and why you are not getting it from your food. Learn how to naturally acquire that nutrient in your diet. (Berry, Which Supplements)

Movement and Metabolism

If you park your car in the garage and do not touch it for three months, you may have difficulty starting it when you need it. Forgive the analogy, but why are some folks amazed that their bodies creak, that they have pain, stiffness, weakness, when they sit on their butts all day?

If you have a body, it needs to move. The phrase "use it or lose it" has never been truer. There is a condition called "learned non-use." (Taub) It means that we learn to not use certain parts of our body and allow other parts to attempt to do the job.

As your regular and consistent activity levels rise, your metabolism adjusts to accommodate the energy costs of the movement. Also, your body gets to begin using those wonderful nutrients you are eating to heal and generate new cells. The movement produces flexibility, agility, and your ability to react. Combined with the nutrients you are consuming, your body can begin reducing inflammation, and your immune system becomes more finely tuned.

How long can you stand up without wanting to sit down? How far can you walk without wanting to take a breather? How much physical work can you do without feeling fatigued? How likely are you to be stiff or achy the next day? When was the last time you ran anywhere? Are you less flexible than you used to be?

These common conditions happen, not because we are getting older, but rather we are getting more sedentary. The body regenerates; there is no reason to assume these limitations are due to wear and tear. It is just learned non-use.

Nearly ten years ago, I told my doctor that my knees were hurting. With the shrug of his shoulders, he said, "They are fifty-year-old knees." Of course, he went on to once again encourage me to lose weight, despite my doing what that nutritionist told me to do. I would have said at the time that my diet was healthy, the occasional indulgence aside. He seemed to be suggesting that my body would naturally wear out, that painful knees were part of middle age, and I could expect more parts to begin to falter.

If finding a fun movement has to this point eluded you, start somewhere, anywhere. You can download a pedometer app for your phone. Forget the ten thousand-step prescription. Simply do more steps tomorrow than today.

Consider learning how to stretch correctly for flexibility. You can find lots of free videos online. Walk more and stretch.

After losing one hundred pounds, my knees stopped hurting. So, my doctor was partially correct. But now my butt hurts when I sit for a long period of time. I invested in cushions, but they only helped for a while. A massage therapist near my office asked me if I used my hands to stand up. He suggested that doing so meant I might have *gluteal amnesia*. He said it was fairly common in middle-aged men. (Wow, so sixty is middle-aged?)

I did a little investigating online. I found a couple of diagnostic exercises to try and I found out; he was right. My butt muscles barely moved when I tried to flex them. My butt has forgotten how to work! Instead, my lower back and quads were doing all the work. I am now engaged in reactivating my glutes and improving my posture. (Frampton) (Ethier)

Your posture, walking, and increasing your flexibility are low-impact ways to start. They may not be enjoyable at first, but they can lead to your finding an amazing activity that you love. When you are ready to explore, consider taking advantage of free classes in your area. There are lots of group classes available, and many will offer you a free session to see if you would like to attend.

You will get a sales pitch after the free lesson. Just do not sign up if you are not sure and, if you do decide to have a go, sign up for a minimum number of classes to make sure you keep liking it. In Pittsburgh there are lots of free opportunities, including Yoga, Zumba, tai chi, boxing, and swimming. There are dance classes, tap, ballroom, belly, salsa, pole dancing, and even twerking! Almost all martial arts classes seem to offer a free class or two.

Remember: real, sustainable activity is about enjoyment and getting good at something, not about burning calories, or necessarily building muscles. Although you will probably do both.

You can hire a personal trainer for a minimum number of sessions. Professional physical trainers not only help people with lifting weights but also with your cardiovascular training, posture, stretching, and even gluteal amnesia! The trainer should discuss your goals, any limiting conditions, and then guide you through a session that might leave you a little sore the next day but feeling good about yourself. The best part about hiring a trainer is the accountability involved. Working with a good trainer will keep you motivated.

If you do not want to spend money on classes or a trainer, there are many things you can do on your own, using instructional videos that are actually free on YouTube. You want to be careful and proceed slowly when going solo because moving the wrong way can actually cause physical damage.

Years ago, when I still paid for a gym membership, my gym offered free workout demonstrations for each machine that novices like me used. Despite the free offer, I saw many people attempting to use machines in an unsafe and incorrect manner. I would occasionally speak up, telling them they were going to hurt themselves and that they should just get the free demonstration. I was nice and respectful in my approach.

Whatever you explore and finally choose, you will probably be pretty bad at it at first. Ask yourself, "Would I enjoy getting good at this?" Notice I did not say "being good at this." You have to enjoy getting good at it. That often means working hard at it.

Having fun often takes real work. My nephew plays college football. Preseason football camp, practice during the season, and staying in shape after the season is over requires hard work. He loves the game and loves getting better at it. That's the key.

Mind and Metabolism

If you tell yourself you cannot do something, you will be right, even if you are wrong. It is called the nocebo effect. If a person believes that a particular medication will not work, it will not. This is the opposite of the placebo effect, when a person believes something will work, and it does, even if there is no scientific reason for it to work.

A major aspect of metabolism that most people do not even consider is the role the mind plays. Back in the beginning of this book, I pointed out that I distinguish between mind-body and brain-body relationships. I have made the distinction throughout this text, but in case you do not remember, let me remind you. The brain-body is fairly mechanical, automatic, and functional. If you pinch me, I feel it, but in order to feel it, the brain and the body must communicate. The mind-body connection incorporates perceptions, beliefs, and emotions. The mind, the brain and the body interact and mutually affect one another. If you pinch me, I feel it, *and* I might get angry or annoyed. I might think you are rude or condescending. I might believe there is something wrong with you, or you are a childish person.

We know, for example, that physical movement can reduce depression. (Archer) By the same token, depressed people are often lethargic. Which causes which? Or do they happen in conjunction? While we know about emotional eating, there is a more subtle relationship among emotions, attitudes, and even thoughts that impact brain-body function.

Some people declare that they do not know what it means to feel full. Surely, their stomachs have been full. If leptin is active in their system, they receive a physical sensation of satiety but do not interpret or identify that sensation as feeling full, so they continue to eat.

Some may feel hunger in response to certain emotions, as we have discussed. Others might experience emotions when tasting certain foods that trigger memories.

We also know, for example, that stress releases hormones, namely cortisol, that can cause us to resist weight loss and even may cause us to gain weight. There are both physical and mental kinds of stress, making the attitudes we hold able to impact metabolism either indirectly or directly.

The mind is powerful and can drive change. Many people have experienced success with weight-loss hypnosis even when it is still considered a matter of overeating and self-control. In fact, I know a lot of hypnotists who basically do portion control hypnosis (suggest eating less or feeling full) and aversion therapy (make certain foods taste fowl) to help clients lose weight. Sometimes it works, at least for a while. There is even a hypnosis program that mimics bariatric surgery as extreme portion control.

Throughout this book, I have given you suggestions for structuring your thoughts in a more productive way by changing "I am" statements to "I feel." We have also looked at our internal monologue as a source of suggestion. We have explored the ideas of intentional and mindful eating. Even the notion that movement should be fun and should be something that a person would enjoy getting good at taps on the mind-brain-body relationship.

These are very gentle forms of self-hypnosis. When I have suggested working through this program with a certified Hypnofasting Program hypnotist, it was to help you manage the mind portion of your experience. If you have been going through this program on your own, consider consulting with a trained Hypnofasting Program hypnotist, especially if you have had difficulty adjusting to the changes we have made. You can find a trained hypnotist on our website, www.hypnofastingprogram.com.

In The Hypnofasting Program, hypnosis private sessions are tailored to support the individual client at the particular stage. (Group sessions are, by nature, less customized.) We may include portion control, but only if it is necessary. Mindful and intentional eating habits tend to take care of portion control, the sensation of feeling full. Controlling the carbohydrates helps reduce carbohydrate hunger and manage sugar addiction so that an individual no longer craves sugar.

Hypnosis works on automatic thoughts, reactions, feelings, and behaviors, which factor into metabolism because they drive how we feel, and how we feel is related to hormonal reactions in the body. Those hormonal reactions in the body can have a strong effect on metabolism, the immune system, our motivations, and our confidence.

Hypnotically, if we think or nurture the attitude that we are starving, our bodies may actually respond by going into starvation mode even when we have plenty to eat. This is why we start our journey by addressing hunger. Your internal monologue, or the way you narrate your life, is critical. Yet again, I will caution you against the phrase "I am hungry." Replace it with "I feel hunger." And then look for the trigger that caused the feeling. It probably was not the need for food. In fact, unless there is a chemical addiction, cravings are like hunger, drawing your attention away from something.

When you tell yourself you cannot eat something, all you think about is eating that thing, and you feel the loss or the absence of that food. You automatically and unconsciously set up a goal to eat that food again as soon as you can and often as much as you can.

As I wrote earlier, if you are fasting until 9 a.m. the next morning, do not tell yourself that you will eat at 9 a.m., but that you can eat any time after 9 a.m. It may seem like just a mental game, but the impact is surprisingly strong. If you mentally plan to eat at 9 a.m., you will be ravenous at that specific time, likely because your brain-body believed you and prepared for it.

Healthy eating attitudes and balanced eating emotions can go a long way in convincing your body to freely use the resources available to it, including, and most importantly, that stored fat that it had been saving for lean times. Remember that from now on, we are choosing to eat intentionally.

Gluconeogenesis vs. Ketosis

We have talked about gluconeogenesis before. It is when your liver runs out of glycogen and begins converting fat stores into glucose. Ketosis happens when your body knows you mean business. Your body can make two different kinds of fuel out of fat. It can make glucose, as in gluconeogenesis. And it can also make ketones, as in ketosis. (Manninen)

While the transition from gluconeogenesis to ketosis can be a bit uncomfortable for some, once the transition takes place, most people feel great, have greater clarity of thought, experience very little hunger, have more energy, and even sleep better.

Prolonged strong ketosis appears to have been associated with the occurrence of kidney stones in a small percentage of people. I had a client who is a nurse bring up this issue. I have not found sufficient studies that indicates that ketosis conclusively caused the kidney stones, but the relationship has been noted.

I am frequently in and out of ketosis, and I have opted to take a cranberry supplement as cranberry has been shown to have preventative properties regarding kidney stones. In any case, the supplement will not harm me, but drinking the actual juice would kick me out of ketosis and likely slow or halt gluconeogenesis. If you are prone to kidney stones, you may want to consult your doctor regarding the use of a cranberry supplement. (McHarg)

Fat Adaptation

As you surf the keto world, you will hear the phrase "fat adapted." The existence of ketones in the blood, urine, or breath does not mean your body is "fat adapted." Your body can use both glucose and ketones for fuel. Often, particularly when following a low-carbohydrate diet, the body is actually using both kinds of energy. When the balance tilts securely toward ketones, and the brain adjusts to using ketones rather than glucose, you are said to be fat adapted. (Sher)

One caveat of fat adaptation is that while you may be burning fat, if your diet is perhaps a bit too high in fat, you will be basically burning the fat you consume. That may be fine if you have obtained your objectives and merely want to maintain a keto lifestyle. But if you still want to lose body fat, you may, at that point, need to cut back just a bit on the fat you consume.

Keto Flu

So far, no one knows why some people suffer flu-like symptoms when the brain-body begins to switch from gluconeogenesis to ketosis. You may have faced them even going low carb. They generally are temporary, lasting only a few days at most. Among people who experience keto flu, the reported symptoms are fatigue, constipation, feeling foggy or unclear, irritability, nausea, or headache. (Campos)

119

I have had a number of clients who experienced it once and then never again. Sometimes a client will call me about it because it has taken place after completing the program stages when they are attempting a longer fast.

You have probably already experienced ketosis with the three staggered OMADs. Some even experienced it at their first OMAD.

A Thirty-Six-Hour Fast

Begin the evening before your busiest day of the week. Finish eating at 7 p.m. or any time you find most convenient. No snacking. Remember to stay hydrated. You already understand that if you were doing OMAD, you could eat any time after that hour the next day. Only, this time, when your OMAD would be complete, you take only a glass of water, perhaps with a bit of lemon or lime, and/or a splash of raw apple cider vinegar. Go to bed early if you need to. You can eat any time the next day after the hour you established. If it was 7 p.m., you can eat any time after 7 a.m.

You can easily make this fast a forty-eight-hour fast by waiting until 7 p.m. Pretty easy if you keep busy.

Do longer fasts frighten you? Remember the bone broth trick the first few times you try it, and soon enough, you will not need the interim boost. If you are working with a hypnotist trained in The Hypnofasting Program, they can help you with both your apprehension and successful strategies to cope with hunger.

You can remain in this stage for as long as you like. Maintain a natural fast of sixteen to eighteen hours daily, and each week either do three staggered OMADs or two thirty-six-hour fasts with a preference for the longer fasts.

Chapter 11
Stage Eight

The Ketogenic Diet

Anytime there is a strange word to identify something, there is a bit of mystery around it. Understanding what the ketogenic diet is will help you distinguish between a low carbohydrate/high fat (LCHF) diet and a ketogenic diet. Keto has become for many just another fad diet, resulting in a plethora of questionable processed food products and gimmicks as well as people embracing the word without understanding what it truly means or bothering to learn about the program they are embracing. They make their decisions based on the recommendations of people who promote themselves, their recipes, their products, and their influence based on a label.

Simply put, all ketogenic diets are LCHF, but not all LCHF diets are ketogenic. A ketogenic diet is designed to consume so few carbohydrates that the body switches to using ketones as its main fuel.

A ketogenic diet consists of extremely reduced carbohydrates, often fewer than twenty grams of net carbs daily. These carbs are usually found in fresh vegetables and rarely, if ever, grains. You may choose to count carbohydrates or "calculate the macros" as many ketogenic dieters do, but that is a matter of your own decision. Unless, of course, you are vegetarian or vegan and have to do those calculations in order to approach a reduced carbohydrate diet.

In its simplest form, it comes down to measuring portions and calculating how many grams of net carbohydrates you are consuming compared to protein and fat. Going beyond a serving or meal, calculating what percentage of your daily diet is dedicated to each macronutrient. Another step or two up, and you are venturing into what Thomas DeLauer calls "biohacking." (DeLauer) DeLauer's take on biohacking seems to be less extreme than others.

For some people, biohacking means experimenting on themselves, tracking all sorts of physiological functions and attributing correlations between them. The thing is that correlation does not indicate causation. That is, just because two aspects follow the same progression, one does not necessarily cause the other to happen and, frankly, false assumptions in individual biohacking adventures could be dangerous.

The hypnofasters who test their blood glucose two hours after a meal are doing a very simplified version of biohacking, but we know that certain foods, based on lots of evidence, cause blood glucose to spike. When we test our blood after eating, we know that something or some of the things we ate were involved in the spike. Despite standards like the glycemic index, some people respond a little differently to different foods. We are merely individualizing the information.

We also track our fasting hours, but we do so to see our progression and to give our body time to use its energy stores, not to learn how many hours of fasting it takes to become fat adapted or to enter ketosis. We are not experimenting on ourselves blindly. We track our activity mostly to keep on track. We are not really biohacking, though some might consider it an extremely mild version.

In Ketosis?

It is not only possible but likely that you have already been in ketosis to some degree. It is more likely to happen after a longer fasting period. I am in mild ketosis after a twenty-four-hour fast. If I fast longer, the presence of ketones increases, but that does not necessarily mean I am burning more fat. It means that I will burn ketones for the energy I need.

There are two common ways of testing to see if you are in ketosis. You can purchase inexpensive, over-the-counter test strips. These should be sufficient while you are on the program. If you choose to follow a strict ketogenic diet, you may consider buying an electronic device, similar to a blood glucose meter, that measures ketones.

Most hypnofasters, during the program, will likely move in and out of ketosis. And if you ever really want to accommodate even some carbohydrates again, you will likely do the same. For our purposes, ketones in our urine is simply a sign that our bodies have begun the process of ketosis, and we are likely burning both glucose and ketones as fuel.

Why Is The Hypnofasting Program Specifically NOT Ketogenic?

I had several reasons to avoid promoting using the term ketogenic to describe The Hypnofasting Program. Although I admit that adherents will most like move in and out of ketosis.

First, it is an exceptionally long jump over a deep chasm to go from eating mostly carbohydrates to fewer than twenty grams a day. I want to help you succeed, not present you with a challenge that many would be unable to sustain.

Second, The Hypnofasting Program is about establishing and maintaining a new normal. Each hypnofaster will determine their level of participation in the program, the degree to which they embrace the changes, and thus decide the extent to which they benefit. It is the job of the consulting hypnotist or coach to point out what those limitations might mean in terms of consequences. Also, many changes are easier to make after others are in place. It is important to understand that an individual's choice is far more sustainable than one imposed by the designer of any program.

After completing The Hypnofasting Program, some may choose to go ketogenic or even completely carnivore. Others might just settle into their new normal and make decisions as they go.

Third, the market has been flooded with what I call keto crap! Keto crap is garbage food, highly processed products for things like keto shakes or snack bars. Many of these make use of artificial sweeteners or manufactured chemical ingredients. Hang around the keto world, and you are likely to eventually buy odd ingredients, expensive supplements, MCT oil, or even exogenous ketones—that is, ketones you eat instead of make yourself. Be a bit wary of any social media influencer whose primary business is selling supplements. Most of them make affiliate-link recommendations for products, and the best among them are transparent about that. But if the clear purpose of their videos is to get you to buy their supplements, be cautious and do your research before pulling out your credit card.

Fourth, I have watched keto influencers go through veritable contortions to avoid carbohydrates and still have what they want to eat. They buy and use ingredients not traditionally used in home cooking but in processed food manufacturing in order to obtain the textures and flavors of processed food. I find this truly baffling. If you are avoiding manufactured foods, buying the ingredients for manufactured foods and making them in your home does not really make them healthier.

Trying to find a truly low-carbohydrate form of pasta is admirable, and the person who comes up with a way of manufacturing it will make a mint, but The Hypnofasting Program focuses on making changes, not on providing ways for people to basically stay the same. Sorry to remind you, but you cannot have your cake and eat it too.

Keto cooks can be a valuable source of inspiration for low-carb recipes. However, filling your pantry with the chemicals used in manufactured foods is just not part of a real, whole food eating strategy. After all, the whole purpose of engaging in this program is not only to lose weight, but also to become healthier and give your body the nutrients it needs to thrive.

I observed the same phenomenon among some vegetarians who will go through equally absurd contortions to eat something that resembles meat. I was a vegetarian for twenty years. My own vegetarian diet relied very heavily on soy products and carbohydrates, and I absolutely attribute my diabetes to my vegetarian, seed-oil diet. When a potential vegetarian client tells me that they want to join The Hypnofasting Program, we have to have a long talk about what they call vegetarian.

Fifth, and finally, The Hypnofasting Program relies on the health benefits of intermittent fasting. Fasting is a critical element. It helps us break free of cultivated grazing and the negative health risk of overstimulating insulin and creating insulin resistance. Even if you are not diabetic, obesity is an aspect of metabolic disease. Often enough, this disease is self-induced because we have been adhering to dietary recommendations that simply do not deliver what they promise.

Many people combine keto with intermittent fasting, but quite a few do not. They assume a low-carb diet, despite the chemical additives, will cause them to be thin. Many also assume they can go keto or even do intermittent fasting for a time and then go back to doing whatever they want. If that sort of promise is what you want, you have been reading the wrong book.

I am not convinced that any diet will result in permanent change. The benefits of the ketogenic diet are limited without the fasting. And the benefits of fasting are limited if you continue eating a high-carbohydrate/low-fat diet, especially if you are feeding your body inflammatory seed oils and chemically manufactured "food."

If you are snacking on keto snacks, you are still triggering insulin even if it is less insulin than eating a bag of potato chips. Going keto is a lifestyle choice just beyond the scope of this program. It is an option some hypnofasters make, and they should be making it based on their learning and research.

Ketoacidosis

In your investigations, you may encounter people attempting to discredit the ketogenic diet. They often point to a condition called ketoacidosis. Ketoacidosis is a serious condition in which extreme production of ketones causes the acidity of the blood to rise to dangerous levels. In his presentation, Dr. Sher points out that the condition of ketoacidosis happens in the *absence* of insulin. Unless you suffer from type 1 diabetes, or your pancreas can no longer produce insulin, you do not need to worry about ketoacidosis. (Sher)

It is unlikely that intermittent fasters at our level will ever approach the ketone levels required for ketoacidosis.

The Winning Hand Fast

In 1977, I was a senior in high school. One of my favorite songs that year was "Brick House" by the Commodores. As I was contemplating an alternative fasting pattern for this stage in The Hypnofasting Program, that song came on the radio. Of course, I sang along, and when I came to the phrase, "thirty-six, twenty-four, thirty-six—oh, what a winning hand!" inspiration struck.

We will take three short-term fasts in a row. The first will be a thirty-six-hour fast. Begin and end as you like, but know that after this fast, you will need an eating window of six to eight hours. After you complete your last meal in that window, conduct an OMAD *plus*, anything over twenty-four hours. Eat a single meal. When you finish eating that OMAD meal, fast for at least another thirty-six hours. Oh, what a winning hand!

Since my moment of inspiration, I have enjoyed this sequence of fasts as my most fun. I hope you will enjoy it.

Joseph A. Onesta

Chapter 12
Stage Nine: The Home Stretch

We have come a long way together. This last chapter focuses on approaching and maintaining your objectives. Stage Nine is dedicated to those last few pounds and pushing through any barriers you might have experienced along the way.

Too Late to Eat

While this is not really part of The Hypnofasting Program, the concept of "Too Late to Eat" proved to be the kick in the pants I needed to attempt even longer fasts. Since then, many clients have employed the same strategy, but I suggest waiting until you are well on your way to your goals and are preparing for the process of settling into your new normal. In any case, you can decide if the too-late-to-eat concept will be useful to you.

My own experience grew out of acid-reflux disease that was made worse when I ate too close to bedtime. Some people like going to bed with a full belly. Not me. Some have difficulty sleeping if they do not have a bedtime snack. I trust you have worked your way around your own idiosyncrasies with your hypnotist.

Most of the time, I am an early-to-bed, early-to-rise guy who is healthy, not so wealthy, but sufficiently wise. Some of the things I read when beginning my own Hypnofasting Program told me that my acid reflux might get worse. That, I am happy to say, has not been my experience. In fact, my dependence on acid reflux medications has been progressively reduced.

Because I already had been avoiding food after 7 p.m., the notion simply carried on into my fasting schedule. This meant that if I did not eat before 7 p.m. I would just go to bed without eating. Most often, I successfully staggered my fasting schedule to finish eating before 7 p.m. But sometimes life gets in the way of the best laid plans.

My natural fast is sixteen to eighteen hours. I occasionally eat more often and regularly fast longer. Keep in mind, a sixteen-to-eighteen-hour natural fast is a feasting, not fasting, day. On my feasting days, I eat two, healthy, good-sized, whole-food meals.

Having that limit of taking my last bite at 7 p.m. was convenient if I forget exactly when I took my last bite. That happened sometimes if I would get home tired or if I fell asleep on the sofa before completing my journal. (Don't judge me. I know it has probably happened to you.) Even if I forget, when I finish eating the day prior, I just default to 7 p.m. I know that I can eat anytime after 11 a.m. I do occasionally eat earlier, and those days are either planned, or are the days that my natural fast is shortened for what I deem to be a legitimate reason.

Sometimes, my friends want to go to a restaurant for dinner, and they, like many people, are late eaters. By the time we order, and the food is brought to the table, it is often after-hours for me. While acid reflux has not bothered me for a long time, I can still use it as an excuse not to eat late. When these dinners are impromptu events, as they often are, I can simply say that I have already eaten. It is not a lie;

we have all eaten at some time, and "I have already eaten" is sufficiently ambiguous.

Longer Fasts

In The Hypnofasting Program, I have guided you through establishing a longer natural fast of sixteen to eighteen hours and walked you through OMAD, OMAD *plus* during three staggered OMADs, thirty-six-hour fasts, and The Winning Hand pattern. We are now approaching the time when we take the training wheels off your fasting bicycle.

You have advanced to the stage of tackling longer fasts. You plan them, or they may just happen.

My first seventy-two-hour fast happened because of a perfect storm of factors, mostly beyond my control. I had planned a thirty-six-hour fast that ended at 7 a.m. I did not feel like eating that early. Since I was to meet a friend for lunch, I decided just to wait. My day was fairly busy, and my friend cancelled at the last minute. Yes, I felt hunger. Yes, I felt disappointment. And yes, I will admit to feeling frustrated. But feeling hunger is not worth going out to a restaurant by myself. Most restaurant food is not usually worth eating. Thus, I decided to wait for dinner. That would be my first forty-eight-hour fast. On the way home, I sat in traffic for several hours as people inched around a collision of several cars on the highway. By the time I got home, it was nearly 8 p.m. It was too late to eat.

The next morning as I was getting ready for work, I did not feel hunger. I had fasted for sixty hours and counting. I also realized that if I were going to eat before dinner that evening, I would need to prepare something to bring to work with me. There was no feeling of urgency, so I did not bother. I adjusted my fast to finish eating before 7 p.m. I planned the meal I would prepare. I took meat out of the freezer and put it in the fridge. I left the house comfortable with fasting for technically seventy-one hours.

From that point forward, I knew I could do it because I had done it before. When we develop skill at eating intentionally and mindfully, we can choose to *not eat* with the same degree of intention and mindfulness. Every time I extended that fast, I made my plan to eat after a certain hour. I never broke that plan despite postponing the next meal several times.

Autophagy

"Autophagy" literally means self-eating, and it describes the process your body goes through when it recycles or "consumes" dead or weakened cells or tissues and uses the resource they provide to make new cells. (Glick)

Though known to exist since the 19th century, Yoshinori Ohsumi won a Nobel Prize in 2016 for his work in understanding the mechanisms of autophagy. Lots of people talk about autophagy, and they sound really authoritative, but when we look at the science, truly little is really understood. Additionally, the mechanisms of autophagy are technical enough to boggle the pedestrian mind.

Cells die all the time. Those cells are, in effect, *consumed*, but it may be nicer to say "processed" by the body. The process happens constantly, and as your body increases in wellness because of your diet and movement changes, that process will likely become more efficient. Autophagy happens normally at a slow rate. Fasts extended beyond twenty-four hours gradually increase the rate of autophagy until the period of nutrient deprivation is over—that is, until the fast is broken. (Maggs, Autophagy)

You cannot really control the process of autophagy. Crunches or sit-ups may tighten the abdominal muscles, but they will not make you lose belly fat. You can encourage your body to use its resources to build muscle in the areas you want. For example, if in losing weight, you discover you have flabby arms, you can use resistance training by lifting weights or using bands to build muscle to fill out some of that loose skin. But doing curls will not tell your body to focus its autophagy on that loose skin.

Autophagy brings with it many potentialities that science has only begun to explore. Some studies are examining the role of autophagy in the reduction of tumors and cancers, for example. But as yet, there does not seem to be an effective way of directing what autophagy does. And actually measuring the effects of fasting on autophagy appears to require starvation levels of fasting. (Pietrocola)

Such levels of fasting are not recommended and not endorsed by The Hypnofasting Program. Starvation levels of fasting can traumatize your metabolism. One of the central tenets of hypnofasting is the establishment of a new normal. Starvation fasting has nothing to do with a new normal.

Autophagy will happen naturally and the longer you maintain your new normal, once you reach it, the more efficient and tailored that autophagy is likely to be. Autophagy is not something we are working toward. It is not necessary to do so.

Until You Reach Your Goal

I do not know how long it will take to reach your goal or if you will change your goal once you reach it. But here are my recommendations to keep you on track.

- Avoid creating patterns of eating behavior. We do not want our brain-body to settle into a new normal before it is time.
- Plan a weekly longer fast. An OMAD or two, or a thirty-six-hour fast or two on a biweekly basis, and in the alternate weeks, perhaps staggered OMADS or The Winning Hand.
- Longer fasts are up to you.
- Maintain an average natural fast of sixteen to eighteen hours on feasting days.

- Eat two or three meals, during your six- to eight-hour eating window.
- Eat intentionally and mindfully until you are full. Then stop.
- Avoid mindless snacking.
- Stay hydrated.
- Move, move, move, and have fun with it.
- Avoid falling into a routine.
- Maintain a low-carb/high-fat diet throughout.
- Stay in contact with your hypnotist for support even if you schedule sessions less frequently.
- If your progress slows down or you reach a plateau, that is, a time when you seem to be in a holding pattern and not making progress anymore, do something to shake things up:
- Try cutting back on fat just a bit. If you are in constant ketosis and you are not losing weight, you may be mostly burning the fat you consume.
- You can reduce your natural fast for a few days and then do a series of staggered OMADs or The Winning Hand.
- You might choose to do a fast longer than you ever have.
- You might stagger your movement and activities.
- You might take a short vacation, relax, have some fun.
- You might try a new or different activity.

When You Reach Your Goal

As you approach your goal, it is time to reconsider how you imagine your forever, your new normal, to look. You will not imagine the same life you might have when you first started this process because nearly everything has changed, including what you want. What sorts of food will remain as part of your regular diet? Will you want to go keto, or will you want to incorporate a bit more carbohydrates?

What about the role of grains, sugar, and fresh fruit in your life? Now that you have a bit of room, where do they fit in?

You should revisit these questions and any others you can think of whenever new information is available and new conditions present themselves. Pay special attention to aspects of this program that you found particularly difficult or objectionable.

What further changes do you intend to make? In your food? In your fasting regimen? In your movement?

What advice would you give to someone considering The Hypnofasting Program and why?

All of the recommendations for settling in to your new normal are similar to the ones I gave you to approach your goal. The only one I exclude at that point is that I am encouraging you to now establish patterns and hold to them for at least a year.

You may, of course, choose to broaden the time between intermittent fasts. A gradual progression from weekly to biweekly to monthly, to every six or eight weeks might be appropriate. Just remember to keep track, and if your measures of success start going in the wrong direction, stop and reverse.

You probably already have started testing what happens if you eat something that you have cut out while on the program. I do that occasionally, but I always do it intentionally and mindfully. Then, and only then, am I able to accurately assess the experience of eating that thing.

To date, I have added only two items to my regular menu. Perhaps once or twice a month, our family protein will consist of fried fish or chicken purchased as take-out. I try to make these at home with low-carb ingredients but even if we buy them in a restaurant, I do not pick off the breading. I know the coating is made of wheat and it was likely fried in vegetable oil. These are rare enough in our diet that I do not overly concern myself. I still check my blood glucose after eating them. There is a rise, but it is not a real spike and is always in normal range.

I continue to do weekly intermittent fasting, usually an OMAD or a thirty-six-hour fast. I occasionally do three staggered OMADs or my new favorite, The Winning Hand.

I will rarely take a bite of my husband's desert. (I am usually disappointed.) I like eating the potato skin after he finishes his baked potato.

More than a year into my program, I visited my doctor and for the second time in a year, my A1c was 5.4 (not even prediabetic). I asked him for a homeostatic insulin resistance test to see how much insulin resistance remained. He refused to prescribe it saying he did not see the value in the test. Since that was the case, I asked him when he would remove the "diabetes" diagnosis from my health record. He seemed shocked at the question and actually wondered out loud if it were even possible. Apparently, he would forever consider me a diabetic.

When I pressed him, he said, *"When you can eat like me."*

I am usually quicker on my feet, but I had no response. Since that moment, I have formulated the answer I would like to give if he were to ever say that again.

Well, Doc, that really depends on exactly what you eat. I don't know if I would want to eat like you, and honestly, if you think the USDA-prescribed low-fat, high-carbohydrate diet is the best nutritional advice, I suspect you are in for a big surprise when you get a bit older.

I wonder if he would get my point.

Epilogue

When I began my own journey, I was completely alone, skeptical, and scared. I worried that it would not work. I was afraid that I would somehow do something stupid and damage my health. It was also quite frightening to learn that my health and wellness were in my hands and were not the sole auspices of my physician.

I, like other "barbarians at the gate," am one of many living success stories. It has been an honor and a privilege to share both my experience and this program with you.

I had several goals in writing this book. Of course, I wanted to share my story and I hoped it would help you. I also wanted to create a practical plan to use with my clients because I wanted to spend more of our valuable time together using hypnosis rather than teaching them the elements of the program. I wrote the book in a way that just about anyone could follow the program on their own, but I hoped most would choose to work with a trained hypnotist and participate in our Facebook group.

If you chose not to work with a hypnotist, I hope the psychological techniques I described helped you. I would still love it if you saw a hypnotist, even just to learn what hypnosis is like and what an invaluable tool it is for both wellness and happiness. Please consider leaving a five-star review for the book.

Your hypnotist should send you a program evaluation form once your sessions conclude. Please take the time to complete it and also share your experience with the program and with others, including your physician. If you do not receive an evaluation form, please feel free to contact me directly at www.hypnofastingsolution.com.

I truly wish you well and hope someday if ever we cross paths, or you would like to write me, that you share your success with me. It would be wonderful to know that this program has helped you. I trust that your life has improved as mine has. Together, let's make the world a healthier, happier place.

Joseph A. Onesta

Supplemental Materials & Sources

Use the words in parentheses from the text to find the corresponding entry. You can download an live-link version of this list at www.hypnofastingprogram.com.

Ali, N., MD (Presenter). (2019, April 3). Presentation: Why LDL cholesterol goes up with a low carb diet and is it bad for health?' [Video file]. Retrieved September 8, 2020, from https://youtu.be/qXtdp4BNyOg

Alirezaei, M., Kemball, C., Flynn, C., Wood, M., Whitton, J., & Kiosses, W. (2010, August). Short-term fasting induces profound neuronal autophagy. Retrieved October 05, 2020, from https://www.ncbi.nlm.nih.gov/pmc/articles/PMC3106288/

Archer, T., Josefsson, T., & Lindwall, M. (2014). Effects of physical exercise on depressive symptoms and biomarkers in depression. Retrieved October 05, 2020, from https://pubmed.ncbi.nlm.nih.gov/25470398/

Avena, N., Rada, P., & Hoebel, B. (2007, May 18). Evidence for sugar addiction: Behavioral and neurochemical effects of intermittent, excessive sugar intake. Retrieved September 16, 2020, from https://www.ncbi.nlm.nih.gov/pmc/articles/PMC2235907/

Berry, K., MD (Presenter). (2017). Which Supplements Should I take? [Video file]. Retrieved 2020, from https://youtu.be/2UCErTNNVXU

Berry, K., MD (Presenter). (2018, August 11). How to Raise Your HDL & Lower Your Triglycerides (NOT what you Think) [Video file]. Retrieved September 16, 2020, from https://youtu.be/FAprJVXq1fE

Berry, K., MD (Presenter). (2018, December 1). Lower BLOOD PRESSURE Naturally (10 Things to Know) 2020 [Video file]. Retrieved September 17, 2020, from https://youtu.be/I4poezuUM5s

Berry, K., MD (Presenter). (2018, December 15). Is Salt Bad for ME??? (Hidden Research) 2019 [Video file]. Retrieved September 17, 2020, from https://youtu.be/1lpH06ely7E

Berry, K., MD (Presenter). (2018, January 14). Counting Calories is Stupid [Video file]. Retrieved September 16, 2020, from https://youtu.be/pMzLXGKNaVg

Berry, K., MD (Presenter). (2018, June 27). 7 Things Your Doctor Got Wrong About Fat [Video file]. Retrieved September 16, 2020, from https://youtu.be/FB4V7Ry1vB8

Berry, K., MD (Presenter). (2018, March 25). KETO Increased Your Cholesterol?? (Here's why It's OK) [Video file]. Retrieved September 8, 2020, from https://youtu.be/-QwD4xoSmRg

Berry, K., MD (Presenter). (2019, August 12). Why Calories Don't Count [Video file]. Retrieved September 16, 2020, from https://youtu.be/KY7f9VAtJD0

Berry, K., MD (Presenter). (2019, January 17). What can you Drink while Intermittent Fasting? (Fast Breakers 2019) [Video file]. Retrieved September 29, 2020, from https://youtu.be/XvKK7xaYVKk

Berry, K., MD. (2019). Lies my doctor told me: Medical myths that can harm your health. Auberry, CA: Victory Belt.

Campos, M., MD. (2018, October 18). What is keto flu? Retrieved October 04, 2020, from https://www.health.harvard.edu/blog/what-is-keto-flu-2018101815052

Center for Food Safety and Applied Nutrition. (2018, October 22). Use of the Term Natural on Food Labeling. Retrieved September 20, 2020, from https://www.fda.gov/food/food-labeling-nutrition/use-term-natural-food-labeling

Charles, D. (2019, May 30). Safe Or Scary? The Shifting Reputation Of Glyphosate, AKA Roundup. Retrieved October 29, 2020, from https://www.npr.org/sections/thesalt/2019/05/30/727914874/safe-or-scary-the-shifting-reputation-of-glyphosate-aka-roundup

Choose My Plate (957834196 745757377 USDA, Trans.). (2020). Retrieved October 01, 2020, from https://www.choosemyplate.gov/

David, L., & Couric, K. (Directors). (2014). Fed-Up [Motion picture on Online reltal]. USA: Atlas Films.

DeLauer, T. (Presenter). (2019, November 11). Calculating Macros & Biohacking for Weigh Loss [Video file]. Retrieved 2020, from https://youtu.be/waNuOaVesIY

Diabetes.co.uk, D. (Producer). (2012, April 12). Low Blood Sugar Symptoms [Video file]. Retrieved September 17, 2020, from https://youtu.be/Coo-zqp3xgE

Dvoskin, R. (2008, April 01). Sweeter Than Cocaine. Retrieved September 16, 2020, from https://www.scientificamerican.com/article/sweeter-than-cocaine/

Ekberg, S. (Presenter). (2019, June 24). Dawn Phenomenon: High Fasting Blood Sugar Levels On Keto & IF [Video file]. Retrieved September 27, 2020, from https://youtu.be/2l80su1zCLc

Ethier, J. (Presenter). (2020, May 17). The Perfect 10 Minute Daily Posture Routine [Video file]. Retrieved 2020, from https://youtu.be/RqcOCBb4arc

Ethier, J. (Presenter). (2020, August 2). How to Awaken Your Glutes [Video file]. Retrieved 2020, from https://youtu.be/rsxKcJVTtUw

Euractive, A. (2012, September 20). French study re-launches GMO controversy. Retrieved September 20, 2020, from https://www.euractiv.com/section/agriculture-food/news/french-study-re-launches-gmo-controversy/

Food & Drug Administration (2019, April 1). CFR - Code of Federal Regulations Title 21. Retrieved September 17, 2020, from https://www.accessdata.fda.gov/scripts/cdrh/cfdocs/cfcfr/cfrsearch.cfm?fr=101.22

Food Revolution, N. (2020, July 31). Uncovering Food Fraud in the Olive and Avocado Oil Industries. Retrieved September 21, 2020, from https://foodrevolution.org/blog/food-fraud-olive-oil-and-avocado-oil/

Frampton, R. (Presenter). (2016). Why Sitting Down Destroys You [Video file]. Retrieved 2020, from https://youtu.be/jOJLx4Du3vU

Fung, J., MD (Presenter). (2016, July 8). The Calorie Deception [Video file]. Retrieved September 16, 2020, from https://youtu.be/5F5o0a4p_3U

Fung, J., MD (Presenter). (2017, May 26). Dr. Jason Fung - 'A New Paradigm of Insulin Resistance' [Video file]. Retrieved 2020, from https://youtu.be/eUiSCEBGxXk?list=WL

Fung, J., MD, & Teicholz, N. (2018). The diabetes code: Prevent and reverse type 2 diabetes naturally. Vancouver, BC: Greystone Books.

Fung, J., MD. (2016). Obesity Code. Vancouver, BC: Greystone Books.

Gammon, C. (2009, June 23). Weed-Whacking Herbicide Proves Deadly to Human Cells. Retrieved October 29, 2020, from https://www.scientificamerican.com/article/weed-whacking-herbicide-p/

Glick, D., Barth, S., & Macleod, K. F. (2010, May). Autophagy: Cellular and molecular mechanisms. Retrieved October 24, 2020, from https://pubmed.ncbi.nlm.nih.gov/20225336/

Gregory, P. R. (2012, July 30). Are One In Five American Children Hungry? Retrieved October 01, 2020, from https://www.forbes.com/sites/paulroderickgregory/2011/11/20/are-one-in-five-american-children-hungry/

Harvard Health, P. (2020, January 6). Glycemic index for 60+ foods. Retrieved September 08, 2020, from https://www.health.harvard.edu/diseases-and-conditions/glycemic-index-and-glycemic-load-for-100-foods

Original date of publication before this update was February 2015.

Hasse, A. (Director). (2012). Edible City: Grow the Revolution [Motion picture on Internet & Premium Channel Viewing]. US: East Bay Pictures International.

Heijmans, B., Tobi, E., Stein, A., Putter, H., Blauw, G., Susser, E., . . . Lumey, L. (2008, November 4). Persistent epigenetic differences associated with prenatal exposure to famine in humans. Retrieved October 02, 2020, from https://www.ncbi.nlm.nih.gov/pmc/articles/PMC2579375/

Houck, B. (2019, April 11). 'Natural' Means Practically Nothing When It Comes to Food. Retrieved September 20, 2020, from https://www.eater.com/2019/4/11/18304951/natural-food-organic-meaning-difference-hormel-meat-lawsuit

Interview: Dr. Ronald Krauss on LDL Cholesterol, Particle Size, Heart Disease & Atherogenic Dyslipidemia [Video file]. (2015, October 16). Retrieved September 8, 2020, from https://youtu.be/7gZt9DQqtZI

Knobbe, C0., MD (Presenter). (2020, June 13). Dr. Chris Knobbe - 'Diseases of Civilization: Are Seed Oil Excesses the Unifying Mechanism? [Video file]. Retrieved September 16, 2020, from https://youtu.be/7kGnfXXIKZM

Lipton, B. H. (2003). The biology of belief. Memphis, TN: Spirit 2000.

Lustig, R., MD. (n.d.). 56 Names of Sugar. Retrieved September 08, 2020, from https://robertlustig.com/56-names-of-sugar/

Magee, E. (2005). Your 'Hunger Hormones'. Retrieved September 04, 2020, from https://www.webmd.com/diet/features/your-hunger-hormones

Maggs, D. (Presenter). (2020, January 7). The pros and cons of intermittent fasting [Video file]. Retrieved 2020, from https://youtu.be/HgB2ogpC6gI?list=PLAp8c94JydGxmHtYxnj4KyQrP74pS-scs

Maggs, D., MD (Presenter). (2020, January 21). Autophagy And Fasting-How To Induce Autophagy For Amazing Health Benefits [Video file]. Retrieved October 5, 2020, from https://youtu.be/eWn83VIZyvs

Manninen, A. (2004, December 31). Metabolic effects of the very-low-carbohydrate diets: Misunderstood "villains" of human metabolism. Retrieved October 03, 2020, from https://www.ncbi.nlm.nih.gov/pmc/articles/PMC2129159/

McHarg, T., Charlton, K., & Rodgers, A. (2003, November). Influence of cranberry juice on the urinary risk factors for calcium oxalate kidney stone formation. Retrieved October 03, 2020, from https://pubmed.ncbi.nlm.nih.gov/14616463/

Nunes, L. (2020, February 25). Sugar vs. Cocaine: The Science Behind Why Sugar is So Bad For You. Retrieved September 16, 2020, from https://brainmd.com/blog/what-do-sugar-and-cocaine-have-in-common/

Parrish, B. (Presenter). (2020, June 28). Dirty Dozen List for 2020- What Fruits and Vegies to Buy Organic vs Conventional [Video file]. Retrieved 2020, from https://youtu.be/7X1z5kjkpTc

Parrish, B. (Presenter). (2019, December 28). Cooking Oil Review At The Grocery Store - Healthy vs Toxic Oils [Video file]. Retrieved September 17, 2020, from https://youtu.be/X1Oe-4qkID0

Parrish, B. (Presenter). (2020, August 27). You're Buying FAKE Avocado Oil - The Great Avocado SCAM! [Video file]. Retrieved 2020, from https://youtu.be/X--2YBI-sn4

Parrish, B. (Presenter). (2020, September 24). You're Buying Fake Olive Oil...Here's How To Avoid It! [Video file]. Retrieved 2020, from https://youtu.be/Hg2-iukG80U

Pearce, R. (Director). (2009). Food, Inc. [Video file]. Retrieved 2020, from http://www.documentarymania.com/player.php?title=Food%20Inc

Pietrocola F, Demont Y, Castoldi F, Enot D, Durand S, Semeraro M, Baracco EE, Pol J, Bravo-San Pedro JM, Bordenave C, Levesque S, Humeau J, Chery A, Métivier D, Madeo F, Maiuri MC, Kroemer G. Metabolic effects of fasting on human and mouse blood in vivo. Autophagy. 2017 Mar 4;13(3):567-578. doi: 10.1080/15548627.2016.1271513. Epub 2017 Jan 6. PMID: 28059587; PMCID: PMC5361613.

Perlmutter, D. (2017). Brain maker: The power of gut microbes to heal and protect your brain - for life. London, UK: Yellow Kite.

Ravnskov, U., Diamond, D., Hama, R., Hamazaki, T., Hammarskjöld, B., Hynes, N., . . . Sundberg, R. (2016, June 01). Lack of an association or an inverse association between low-density-lipoprotein cholesterol and mortality in the elderly: A systematic review. Retrieved September 16, 2020, from https://bmjopen.bmj.com/content/6/6/e010401

Sher, D. (Presenter). (2018, June 22). Dr. Doron Sher - 'Understanding Ketones' [Video file]. Retrieved 2020, from https://youtu.be/z7Lx-GHGMBc

Shmerling, R. H., MD. (2019, February 21). Sweeteners: Time to rethink your choices? Retrieved September 20, 2020, from https://www.health.harvard.edu/blog/sweeteners-time-to-rethink-your-choices-2019022215967

Strawbridge, H. (2020, February 03). Artificial sweeteners: Sugar-free, but at what cost? Retrieved September 20, 2020, from https://www.health.harvard.edu/blog/artificial-sweeteners-sugar-free-but-at-what-cost-201207165030

Symptoms of Low Blood Sugar. (2018, July 25). Retrieved September 04, 2020, from http://www.healthlinkbc.ca/health-topics/aa20831

About the Author

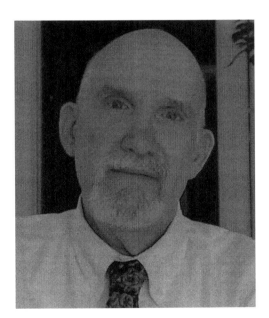

Joseph A. Onesta is a clinical hypnotist in Pittsburgh, Pennsylvania. He has had a number of successful careers. His choices have always reflected a dedication to empowering others to reach for and achieve a fulfilling life.

In 1986, having earned a master's degree in English he moved to the Bronx, NY, where he taught Academic English as a Second Language helping students acquire the language skills needed to earn an American college degree.

In the 1995, while still teaching part-time, now at Los Angeles City college, he developed an internationally recognized social, educational, and recreational program for AIDS Project Los Angeles at the height of the AIDS Pandemic. It was there that he was first exposed to clinical hypnosis and saw what wonders the practice of hypnosis could provide.

His next project was leading a team of talented public speakers and financial educators for Consumer Credit Counseling of Los Angeles. He and the team educated some 20,000 people annually on effective personal finance strategies.

After some 30 years in higher education with some brief forays into the not-for-profit world, he and his husband decided to move to be near Joseph's family in Pittsburgh. Harkening back to his time at AIDS Project Los Angeles, with the support of his husband, Joseph pursued certification in clinical hypnosis. He graduated with honors from the Hypnosis Training Institute in Newport Beach, CA. He is certified by the International Medical and Dental Hypnosis Association (IMDHA), the American Council of Hypnotist Examiners (ACHE) and the International Certification Board of Clinical Hypnotherapy, (ICBCH) where he is also a certified hypnosis instructor. He is a regular featured speaker and hypnosis educator at professional conferences.

Joseph may be contacted at www.hypnofastingsolution.com.

Made in the USA
Columbia, SC
07 March 2021

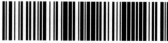